# arms

# arms

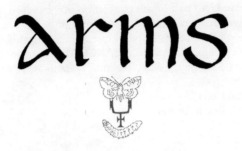

## Madeline Sonik

**Symbols by Alison Skelton**

**Nightwood Editions**
*Roberts Creek, 2002*

**Nightwood Editions**
R.R. #22, 3692 Beach Avenue
Roberts Creek, BC
Canada V0N 2W2

THE CANADA COUNCIL | LE CONSEIL DES ARTS
FOR THE ARTS | DU CANADA
SINCE 1957 | DEPUIS 1957

Cover photograph by Kristin Sweetland
Author photograph by Eric Henderson
Edited for the house by Silas White
Printed and bound in Canada

We gratefully acknowledge the support of the Canada Council for the Arts
and the British Columbia Arts Council for our publishing program.

**National Library of Canada Cataloguing in Publication Data**

Sonik, Madeline, 1960–
  Arms

  ISBN 0-88971-181-X

  I. Title.
PS8587.O558A75 2002     C813'.6          C2002-910268-5
PR9199.3.S573A75 2002

*This work is dedicated to my partner, Eric, and our daughters, Madeline and Dyana.*

# Contents

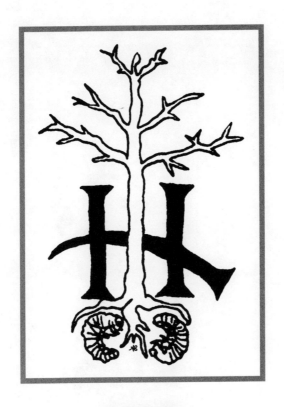

**ARMS**

When his eyes got all red-rimmed-raging, stuck out of his face like bloody ledges, dissected us with the blunt beam of his bruised and drowning pupils, my brother and I buried ourselves.

Our mother continued bitching. She bitched all day anyway. Bitched like spew. Bitched in the bathtub, over brown ivory walls, bitch, bitch, bitch, bitch into the kitchen sink, the roasting pan. She bitched till her glasses cracked, bitched till the cherry lesions of eczema on her hands and cheeks oozed.

We crawled under bedclothes, under beds. We made ourselves infinitesimally small, we turned to powder, slipped into hardwood cracks, stayed like that so long we were afraid to come back. The house was in ruins. Broken-limb light fixtures. Craters the size of an elephant's ass. The couch, torched. The television, imploded. Beef flaming on the back porch like napalm. Tiptoeing past his lopsided La-Z Boy, we noticed our mother's nose plastered to the wall.

"Aw I want you to do is caw. Caw . . . that's aw. Is that too buch to as?"

The voice was not coming from the nose.

"I cook and clee for you . . . you bonster. I wash your

shitty underwear you botherfucker . . . you can't eben caw?"

The voice was coming from somewhere on the floor.

"Eben when I tell you how ibportant it is to be . . . eben when you know . . . you still don't caw . . ."

We carefully lifted our feet, sailed through the debris of dangling door frames, moved out into the cool green night like refracting moons.

My brother took my hand. Our flesh melting together.

"How long?" I asked him.

"Don't know . . . better wait."

The forest behind our house lives at night. All dark creatures of day that hide or cower away from the presbyopic sun take flight. The spruce and hemlock bow, the bracken ferns relax their rigid hold.

We slide down seamless paths of fallen needles, brown as moth wings, moist as sex. We talk of dropping deeply into each other like sinking stones in canyons. It's still too early to leave.

We lie beneath sappy shelters when we tire, enclose each other in thick, pink laces of arm, perfectly content.

At dawn, he nudges me. Dim stars disappear. "Let's not leave," he says. "Let's keep going."

At home, mattress-sized bandages reel across wrenched walls, dislocated doorways push themselves straight, glass continents that have broken free from wounded windows sweep themselves out of existence.

"We should go back," I say. "Everything will be okay."

Our mother peels her nose off the wall, sticks it back on her face with glossy friction tape we are meant to ignore.

"Something smells," she says tentatively, practicing her nose, and then more boldly: "What the hell stinks?"

He has shrunk. His eyes smaller than split peas, his mouth tiny and puckered as a rat's tit. He hangs over the morning newspaper, crippled chair smouldering.

"I don't smell a god-damned thing," he says. "And you?" he asks, folding his wiry body towards us. "Do you smell a god-damned thing?"

Smudge rolls off the slow-cooking couch like wet kindling. Small piles of putrefying entrails puddle at his feet.

"Smell? What smell?" my brother says. "I don't smell a thing."

Our mother adjusts her nose. She inhales again, this time like an expanding furnace. "Don't tell me something doesn't stink. I can smell, can't I? I have a nose! What are you all trying to do? Drive me crazy? Make me think I don't smell something when I do? What's wrong with you?"

He folds his paper on his lap. His curved, flaccid spine has become ramrod stiff, his shallow eyes ringed planets, his shoulders swell, his face distends. My brother whispers, "Run!" He hurls himself beyond the splintering porch stairs. My heart jumps in my throat. I spin to follow him. Melting linoleum rises under my feet. I vault past my sniffing mother.

"No one gives a damn about all the work I do," she's saying. "You all just act like I'm the fucking cleaning lady. You all just think you can make any god-damned stinking mess you please."

I dive for the trembling door. The walls undulate like collapsing rubber. I see my brother, bloodless, turn as he reaches the threshold of the forest. I see him drop to his knees, dig the leaf-strewn earth with cupped hands. In a moment he disappears.

Before I'm able to join him, the explosion occurs. Heaving plasterboard and corrugated metal discharge like shrapnel. Two twirling shingles lop off my arms. I kick the dirt back frantically with my feet, hoping to find him before the next detonation. I throw my scorched body into the cool, open ground.

Severed halves of an earthworm, we meet. I crawl into his flesh.

"Where are your arms?" he whispers.

"Lost," I say, trying not to sob.

He is stoically silent, heroically grave. He contains me in his sausage-casing skin.

"We aren't going back there," he says.

I'm embarrassed that I whimper.

The air beyond us fills with flashes of violet, the unmistakable scent of carbon.

"Christ," my brother says simply, and then another blazing light overloads the sky, scorching the dank earth above us.

"We're going to move. Now!" my brother says, scratching, then gnawing the pungent black soil.

I think of my lonely arms, wrapped in a tree, snagged in thorny rose bushes. My eyes are lead marbles, and I blink to hold them in.

"We'll come back later and find your arms," my brother says gruffly. He burrows us easily through dense sheets of moss. We slip through tangled roots, descend beneath impenetrable rocks, move above the din of anxious chattering beetles.

*Arms*

When we no longer feel the warmth of searing skies, we emerge in the middle of nothing, like deep-sea divers, breaking thin horizons. The stars, urgent flares.

"You okay?" my brother asks.

"I think so," I say, ashamed and naked without arms.

"We can go back and look in the morning," he offers. "First thing." But when the pink dawn peels the night clean, my brother leads us deeper into the forest. A thin and winding trail possesses him. It is filled with jagged curves, fallen trees and the lichen-covered frames of children.

We are mesmerized, enthralled. A young armless girl, tangled in the brutal arrowhead wire of glistening ivy, stares with dead eyes.

If I had arms, I would embrace my shaking body. I would lift my hands to my face, cover my eyes, hold the aching scream in my mouth.

"Don't look," my brother says. "It's nothing."

But I can't pull myself away. I can't stop screaming. "You said we'd go back. You promised we'd find them."

My brother's face is empty. He moves dismissively forward. "We can't," he says.

"My arms!" I scream. "My arms!" I want my voice to stab him. I want my voice to impale him on a tree.

"If we'd left the night I said, you'd still have your god-damned arms. Now you're going to have to just make do without them."

If I had arms, I would slap him with my hands, pinch him with my fingers, twist them over his throat till he choked and did what I said.

"You bastard! You motherfucker! My arms!" I scream.

He walks ahead of me, faster than I can keep up. Without arms, I'm afraid to run.

"Wait for me!" I yell.

He slows a little, his chin and nose stonily tilting forward, his hunched shoulders negligent. "Move it, then."

He is still ten feet ahead of me. Without arms, I'm off balance, clumsy. I slip over mossy rocks and stones. "Come back here. Come back here and help me!"

But the wind decapitates words. It opens vowels like knife blades. We walk for miles without him hearing. When he stops, my voice has vanished.

He watches me approach the clearing where he sits on a tree stump. His eyes are like small scars.

"I don't want to hear any more about your god-damned arms, understand?"

He points at a battered, abandoned shack. Tall, green,

wasted boards tapped together with jagged pegs, worm-hole windows. "Get in," he says.

I slide through the narrow opening, pull myself across the fractured floor on my belly, twist to my side. There is a smell of flourishing mould, ravenous insects, rot.

I rock back and forth, gaining momentum to sit, then kneel and stand. My head brushes fragile beams, my face absorbs cobwebs. I lean against the dark walls so my eyes and mouth are level with the bright, open holes.

"I still want my arms," I call. "Do you hear me?"

I watch my brother begin to expand. "I'll go back and get your god-damned arms if you can't live without them," he says.

He rises, pitches a handful of sharp stones at the shack. I press my eye tight to the hole wanting to see him retreat, but he is like a streak of silver fuse, moving faster than fire, igniting the forest floor with speed, moving away from me, moving away and forward, more and more deeply into the forest.

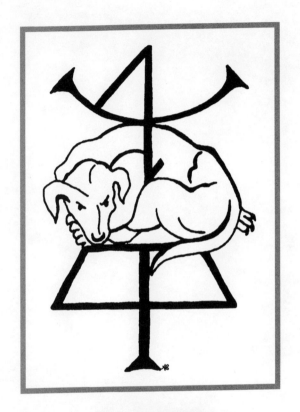

**HUNGER**

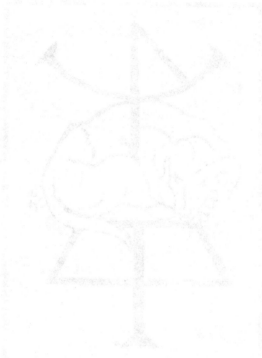

What is at the end of the forest? Where does the forest end? It is like an island, disappearing into gravel, into tarmac streets, into tall glass buildings, into malls and parking lots, dust and lights, people walking, broken bottles, sidewalks, stop signs, words on every corner.

He is like a small animal, sap stains and perspiration decorate his shirt, his hair stands attentive as pine needles. There is something he has left in the forest.

"Kiss me!" a girl shouts. He looks at her. Her skin is the colour of walnuts.

There are people everywhere, walking and walking, dogs running by themselves, shitting, cars screeching and honking.

He looks at the girl. She is just a little girl. There is a man selling french fries on the street, a woman in a short black skirt carrying the heel of one shoe, a midget crying.

The little girl peels a kiss off her lips like wax. She sticks it on a building and walks away. He moves quickly to grab it before anyone notices, before it falls to the ground. He stuffs it in his mouth, but it doesn't taste good, it isn't sweet. It doesn't fill him.

He thinks he will go back into the forest, travel straight

across it, eat berries from the trees, but now he cannot find his way.

A man in a car pulls up and offers him food. There are raw hunks of red meat in the back seat. The cardboard air freshener hanging from the radio knob does nothing to mask the smell of blood.

"Get in," the man says. "What's your name?"

He doesn't know his name. He isn't sure.

"Could it be Ralph?" the man chuckles. "How about Joe?"

Joe is what the man decides to call him.

"Hey Joe, whatdayaknow?"

Joe says nothing.

"They call me Horace," the man says, extending five chunky fingers that jerk at Joe's hand.

The man is wearing a cowboy hat, he has spurs on his heels. "You just get into town, Joe?" he asks. His stomach touches the steering wheel. His smile is broader than a horseshoe.

The smell of blood makes Joe drool, then feel sick. He pretends he doesn't see the meat.

"You do for me, I'll do for you," the man says. His fingers like small pork sausages come to rest on Joe's curving shoulder.

The man drives past stores, past people and street light poles, he drives in stops and starts, bursts of forward motion. Cars and trucks nudge ahead, buses turn right and left, but the man continues up the black patchy street, along one solid yellow line.

Everywhere buildings crawl into the sky like rockets on patches of grass and cement. The road is airless. The car's belly brushes the earth.

"Here's where I live!" the man says, veering sharply left, rolling down a concrete ramp where metal spikes, sharp as spears, rise and fall like chewing teeth.

There are axe-blades on his walls, pockets of dank emptiness, kettle holes the size of heads where timid lizards slip away and out of sight.

There are no windows here, no doors that close, chambers hemorrhage without restriction through ballooning tunnels.

"It ain't much, but home!" the man says, removing his hat, tossing it like a dish into the darkness.

Joe stands with his back against bars, something liquid drips in his collar, runs past his spine. In this blackness he recalls the forest and touches his body for some clue of what it was he'd hoped to find.

The man leads him past rocky fangs into a scalloped depression, rattles a chain at the threshold. "Guest room," he laughs. "Make yourself comfortable."

Joe stumbles blindly into the hollow, inhaling bloody meat. His pupils are swallowed by lightlessness. The small hairs on his body sway like feelers.

"You adjust," the man assures, locking a chain around his throat. Silence rings like the ripple of drops in a pool. The meat is cold and delectable, its juice salty. Joe tears it from the bone, his tongue and teeth embracing its sinewy rawness.

"Steady on, Joe," the man's voice calls. "Don't make yourself sick."

But Joe can't stop, can't take enough in, his hunger devours him, makes him shake the meat in his aching teeth until it rips, makes him gnaw and chew and suck until his body swells with a low and sonorous growl, and he retches, bringing all of it back.

He cannot see what he's done, but in that moment feels such shame that even in this impenetrable darkness he hopes to find a place to hide. All around, the smell is warm and sour, his stomach rolls, and again he thinks of the forest, of pine nuts and blackberries, and wonders why he left.

He sleeps then, but doesn't know he sleeps, because the

darkness is everywhere, his eyes have lost their feeling, and when he wakes, he has no knowledge of his waking, for both in sleep and wakefulness he consumes the flesh the man brings.

And then comes a sharp pain in his thigh. His naked thigh? Is he dressed or naked? His hands lose their ability to say, his eyes have withered useless, and before long he wonders if it is pain he's feeling or if it's something else.

The man comes and goes, comes and goes, like a train pulling in and out of a station, rumbling along, coughing his presence.

"Once, there was something in a forest," Joe begins. He would like to tell himself a story. He would like to comfort himself. But those words, did he speak them aloud? Did they rip past his lips without his hearing? He wouldn't like the man to have them, he wants them for himself.

Gristle stretches in his mouth like rubber, splintered bones release their chunky marrow. Is it pain? Just one more mouthful and then he will stop and think, then he is sure he will know.

Chains rattle. His chains? He pulverizes another thick ropy bone. He has been here long enough. He has been here too long already.

"I once owned a dog," the man says. His voice falls from the walls like an avalanche. "The best friend you could imagine."

Joe waits for his meat. He's restless now because the man does not bring the meat as he used to, the man talks too much.

"Dog went everywhere with me, did everything I told him."

Joe would like to tear the man apart. Sometimes he thinks he might if he can find him in the darkness, if he doesn't hurry with the meat he just might shred him to nothing.

"I used to feed Dog and take care of him, and of course Dog repaid me in kind . . ."

The unmistakable slap of meat hitting stone excites Joe. His nose runs, his mouth secretes saliva. He hunts for his prize, relishing the thought of that first bite, and then something in his thigh: a needle? a sharp rock? a feather? He doesn't know, he can't even be sure enough to guess. The meat is cool, tough, moist, he pulls it apart neatly, his teeth crush and churn it, but as he eats, he knows there is not as much as there used to be; the man does not bring as much.

Before long, Joe is hungry. Sometimes he thinks he hears

the man, but no meat comes. He strains his neck, strains his shoulders to listen. He wonders if the man can see him in the darkness, if the man stands watching him.

One day, when he thinks the man is there watching, he shouts: "I can be a dog!"

When the man brings meat next, there is more than Joe can eat all at one time. He drags some off, collects stones around it, keeps it safe for himself. He touches it, licks it, just to make sure he lies with his face over it.

The man starts bringing big hunks of meat, whole sides of animals that he drops like felled trees.

Joe jumps up. He gnaws at the irresistible food. He eats much more than he thinks he can hold, and still there is always more to hoard.

The man says, "Good Joe," and tells him he'd like him to bark.

Joe does what the man says. If he had a tail, he would wag it. If he had a snout, he would try to find the man's hand and nuzzle it. It's a game. He can play a game, and soon there will be no need for this game anymore. Soon, Joe thinks, he will no longer need the man.

The man pats his head, his voice trails away, down into different chambers.

Joe buries the meat and bones he can't eat, covers them with loose stones, with clumps of earth and curls above them feeling large.

When the man finally comes to take him away, he doesn't want to go. He digs at his small hill of meat as if he believes he could enter it. The man chuckles softly, he pulls at Joe's chain. "Today's graduation day, Joe." He almost sings.

Joe pulls back on the chain. "It's only a game," he reminds himself, and then, "I could shred this man to dust with my teeth."

The man yanks forward hard loose stones and old excrement scatter. Joe loses his grip on the hill.

"Don't fuss, dog," the man says, dragging him over sharp fingers of rock, through slippery creases of moist stone, into archways where thin trickles of light ricochet, stinging his eyes.

The man tightens the chain. Joe tries to cover his burning eyes. "Move, dog," the man says, and boots Joe in the rear.

Joe flounders in the light. He can see nothing ahead. His eyes stream tears. He bumps into walls, trips over stairs, but the man continues tugging.

"Good dogs do as they're told," the man murmurs.

Joe nips the air. He would rip the man apart if he could find him.

The man kicks Joe again, he kicks until Joe moves forward and up. A long series of cold cement stairs bring Joe to a place of more intense and punishing light. The man drags him into a dream, he drags him into a nightmare, he seals a heavy metal collar around his neck, removes his chain. "A training collar," the man calls it. "A collar to help a bad dog become good."

Joe chokes under the pressure of the collar. His eyes burn as if they've been bathed in acid. His throat is collapsing, breaking in, his breath disappearing.

"The more you panic," the man tells him, "the worse it's going to be."

Joe's fingers reflexively reach for the collar, but slide off its slippery chrome. If only he could pry his fingers underneath the tight collar, break its seal, he would attack the man, put an end to his games. He would run back to the forest, live under the shelter of trees, eat seeds and berries and sweet honeycomb.

The man boots Joe again. His spurs spin and catch. Joe tumbles through a doorway. His swollen eyes stream rivers, his contracting throat closes.

When he wakes, he isn't sure where he is or what has happened. The light no longer blinds him. He touches his body with his hands, touches his throat, his collar. All around him he is aware of light, of white walls, of windows. All around there is air.

He pulls himself to his feet, feels the familiar sensation in his thigh. He is wearing ragged, rotting clothing, yet through a rip he can see a deep, bloody sickle-shaped gash.

The man is nowhere in sight. He has not brought meat. Joe creeps tentatively about the empty room listening, sniffing. His churning stomach empty. He touches the white door, then presses his ear against it, finally, cautiously, pushes it.

Beyond, there is a spacious living room. A television set that covers one entire wall, a long, snaking, cream-coloured settee. Everywhere, there are tinted windows extending from floor to ceiling, the city swimming out of reach.

For a moment, Joe is unable to move. He is afraid of being so high and wants to get flat to the ground, to crawl on his belly, but then he sees the way out. A door at the end of the room.

He skids across the slick-tiled floors, topples a table and lamp that crashes at his feet making him yowl and stumble. He grabs the door handle, twists it like a rag, bolts forward but is forcefully thrown back as the collar grips his neck – like electrical fingers. Again, his throat collapses, his windpipe shuts. Even his reflexive screams can't emanate beyond his suffocation.

"Bad dog," the man says from somewhere behind.

Joe wants to stand, he wants to look fierce, but his body writhes on the cool tile floor, as if it's no longer his.

"Bad dogs don't eat," the man says, and for days Joe is locked in his small white room aching with hunger.

There are other dogs. Joe can hear them snapping and chewing outside his prison. He can smell their food, smell their bodies, and he tries to imagine the most succulent, tender pieces of meat for himself. When he is finally freed, the man introduces him to the others.

They are big, ugly, unfriendly. "We don't want you in our pack," the head dog snarls.

"There's strength in numbers," the man chuckles. "This new dog will make you stronger."

"If you put him in our pack, we'll kill him!" the head dog threatens.

"If you kill him," the man says, "none of you will eat."

The dogs drool over their slippery meat, they growl and fight with each other, nip and yelp.

"Don't let the new dog have any," the head dog orders when the man leaves. Another dog viciously bites Joe's arm.

"Why don't we eat him?" the dog says. "We can pretend we don't know where he went."

"The man will know," the head dog says.

Joe fights for a piece of meat, for one small, tough mouthful. There is not as much as the man used to bring for Joe, not as much as Joe had collected and hid away for himself.

Other dogs knock him away from their banquet, they kick him with their feet, slap him with their hands, punch his weak, hungry stomach into his backbone with their fists.

He crawls along the floor, pulls himself away from their hatred, their danger. He thinks of the man, feels a sudden sharp and gouging pain in his wounded thigh; maybe if he plays the game the man will save him.

The man lounges on his long white couch, he has taken off his pointed boots, his toes are as naked and pink as a litter of newborn rodents.

"Come to your master, Joe," he says. His voice is compassionate, friendly, kind. As much as he hates the man, if Joe had a tail he would wag it.

"I had a dog once," the man begins. "Oh, not like those

other dogs, a special dog, a dog I could really count on." He stretches across the couch, pauses, as if he expects Joe to say something, and then continues.

"He was a real friend, do you know what I mean? A dog you could really talk to, one that understood."

Joe sits on the floor at the foot of the couch; he wonders what to say or do, if anything will make a difference.

"But of course," the man says, "you don't care about that. You only care about yourself, about the meat."

The wound in Joe's thigh twinges like a bare wire, his stomach moans to be filled. "I can care about you," Joe says, "I can understand."

The man's eyes fill with ripe tears, he reaches into his pants' pocket and delivers a small round cake of the most tender meat to Joe. "You mustn't say anything to the others about this," he whispers.

Joe eats the meat quickly before the man has a chance to take it back. The flavour dissolves before it's been anticipated.

"Now be a good dog, Joe, lick my feet."

Joe looks at the man's bare, curling toes, feels a knot tighten in his plaintive stomach. If he licks the man's feet, there will be more food; if he refuses, he will starve.

He approaches the man's feet as he would approach

poison, tilts his head forward, holding his body back. He tries to think of things, other things, anything that will make this experience less grotesque. The man's toes wriggle, Joe can see balls of fuzzy white lint in between.

"Wash my feet, Joe," the man coaxes, "just like Dog used to, then you'll be my special dog."

Joe thinks of the meat, the mountains of meat that arrived in the darkness. He licks the man's toes, imagining meat.

"More gently, Joe," the man commands, "more softly . . . more like a friend."

Joe thinks of the blood in the toes, of their salty pinkness. He can do this. He can lick the man's toes, he can become his special dog, and one day he will bring this game to an end.

He is rewarded with food, great quantities of the best meat and praise, and given a soft place at the bottom of the man's bed at night. For days he sits by the man, watches TV. The other dogs hate him. They all sleep on the same hard floor in the same bare room, they all fight for the same meat.

The man shouts and kicks at the others. He sends them out for hours at a time. When they arrive back, they are always starving and exhausted. Some nights, the man doesn't give them food. The head dog snarls at the man, and Joe can see he would tear him apart if he could.

Joe licks the man's feet when he takes his pointed leather boots off. He licks past sloping bunions, over hard, rugged corns. He licks between toes, on the smooth balls of the man's feet. He knows he is a good dog, knows he will be fed.

In time, the man speaks again about his old companion, Dog, about the special things Dog did for him.

"When I was feeling down," he tells Joe, "Dog would always make me feel better."

There are special things he asks of Joe. Things to make him laugh. Sometimes he dresses Joe in a clown's suit, sometimes he throws pies in Joe's face; some nights, when Joe is sleeping, he drenches him with buckets of cold water.

The meat is always plentiful and sumptuous, always tender and juicy, always accessible, yet Joe continues feeling hungry. The wound in his leg continues aching. At times it feels as if someone were driving nails into his thigh. He tries not to think too much about it, tries not to think at all, but the pain stings his memory and he whimpers in his sleep.

"I need a happy dog," the man tells him, "a bright, cheerful, carefree dog."

He shows Joe pictures in a magazine: shelties and corgis.

Smiling blue-eyed dalmatians tied up like presents, with dangling ribbons at their throats.

"This is what I want you to be," he says to Joe, "a happy tail-wagger." He clips the picture of the dalmatians out and tapes it to his bedroom wall.

When the man sleeps, Joe limps soundlessly to the dressing table and peeks at his own unhappy reflection. His small eyes sink miserably into his doughy face. His meagre nose glistens with grief. Pain shoots through his wounded thigh like a hook. His mouth is a slot of suffering.

He tears the picture of the dalmatians from the wall and consumes it, pisses over the man's doggie magazines, shits on the bedspread.

The man beats him with a belt when he wakes. "I should have known you'd turn out bad like the rest," he hollers.

Joe cowers and snarls. His eyebrows flatten and crease. "I'm not a dog!" he shouts. The raw and oozing gash on his thigh throbs to the beat of his hectic heart. "You can't make me a dog. I'm going back . . . back . . ."; but he can't remember where he came from.

The man kicks him into the kennel room. Joe skids across the slippery, stinking floor like a piece of light furniture. The other dogs, alarmed, scatter uncertain at first what to make of the commotion.

"Back!" Joe yelps. "Back, back, back," aching and frustrated, trying to recall where in the world it is he must go now.

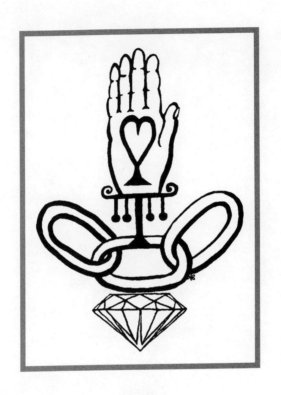

ZO

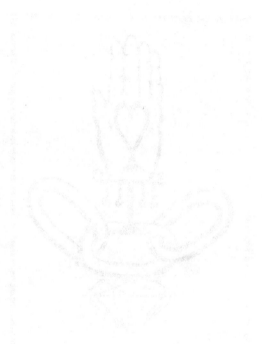

**Z**o is head dog, strong dog. His body's hard, rigid as steel. He does not quail like the others. He does not flee. This fat dog, spilling and skidding into the room so sudden, makes no trouble for Zo. He causes no sweat to break.

Zo stands, all in one piece, not even a twitch, watching this soft white dog twirl on the ground. The man screaming and hollering, while all the rest of us try to look invisible, pushing flat against the wall like glass.

We all say we aren't afraid of that man. We all say he's the biggest motherfucker around, but we all scat when he comes, just like we never say anything.

When we see this man, what we see is his pointed boots. These points, they have silver tips, and these boots, they have spurs. We also see this man has a thick, unfriendly belt. This belt, it has a buckle, and this buckle, it breaks skulls.

If you don't do what the man likes, he beats you. He's got chains too, and electrical collars that lock round your neck. He can zap you so your body doesn't know if it's laughing or dead, so your throat shuts closed like a scab, so all night long you're watching yourself from the ceiling, wondering if it's ever going to be safe to come back down.

Sometimes your mind says you don't want to come back. Sometimes you know it's better to die. Other dogs drag you away then, just like he says, drop you into his big black pit. What he does to you next, no one knows.

This fat white dog, whimpering and shivering on the floor in front of Zo, thinks he knows everything. He's slept on the man's bed, lived in the man's armpit like a flea, now at last the man has flicked him out. He is homeless, friendless, afraid of us and what we might do to him. He is a simpering ass-licker, trying to win Zo with his crumpled, spineless secrets. But Zo is not easily won. There are few things Zo doesn't know, and nothing this cur can teach him.

Zo's lips slide over his strong sharp teeth. His nose wrinkles like peeling wallpaper. This fat white dog cowers, he quakes, not knowing if Zo is angry or pleased, not knowing if Zo will let him live long enough to beg for his life.

Zo laughs from his belly. His laugh is like thunder. He laughs, and the rest of us laugh too. Then Rab dog stops laughing and asks if he can have this dog's heart. All our laughing stops then, and this fat quivering worm of a dog tries to shrink away, to disappear.

"My little friend," is what Zo calls him. "You wouldn't take my little friend's heart," he says to Rab dog.

Rab's eyes are crazy spirals. Drool pulls from his aching mouth like tight string. "Yes, I would. I would take his heart."

"Heart, heart, heart," shout Eta, Mat and Nol. "Let Rab have his heart."

Lee, Ot and me stay quiet. We think maybe Zo might let us draw first blood.

The man watches through his mirrored window. We don't see his face, but we know he's there.

"What kind of a heart do you think my little friend has?" Zo asks Rab.

"A fat heart," Rab says, biting his hungry lip. "A pampered, juicy, bloody heart."

The others howl their approval. The fat dog passes out.

"Look what you've done to my little friend," Zo laughs. "Now if you take his heart, he won't know."

We all laugh with Zo. Rab laughs more than he should.

The man's breath grows louder, unsteady. He wants Rab to take the heart.

Zo touches the air with his tongue. He smiles so the eyes in his head crawl out flat, twists his neck, looks through the mirrored glass. He will not give the heart to Rab. He will not give this dog to us.

Eta, Mat and Nol whine and argue. Lee and Ot snarl and snap. The man will bring no food now. The man will make us starve. But Zo is chief dog, and even if the man brings no food, we will not eat this fat white dog.

Later, he is Joe dog, and is clumsy and breathless when he climbs over fences and crawls through the windows of rich people's homes. He cannot carry much, he does not know where to look for money and jewellery, but goes straight to the refrigerator until Zo boots him in the groin, then he falls on the floor.

"Worthless crap," Zo calls him, Rab takes chunks from his hind. Joe dog whimpers like something dying. Eta begs Zo to eat this dog now. We know he is afraid that Joe dog will be wasted, that he will curl up, rot away to nothing, but Zo says "No," he slings sacks of money at Eta, he dumps golden jewellery from drawers, kicks Joe's wounded ass into action. "You want to live, fat dog?" he asks.

His breath is hot, stinking, solid like wood. We know that Joe dog doesn't care. We know that Joe dog wants to leave his body, rest in the ceiling, never come down, but Zo scares him into living, makes him afraid to die. This dog's feet slip and scatter, his paws gather jewellery into his sack, his wobbly arms stretch like loose rubber, he works himself to an exhausted sweat. He drags his full sack with both hands, he gnaws his sack, dragging it with his teeth. Joe dog, the weak dog, can barely move his sack to the door, but soon, if he lives, he will be strong.

The man waits in his bloody automobile. He looks in his mirror, digs at his teeth. We dogs pick the house clean like a carcass, we leap out the windows, sail over hedges, twist past the fence. Joe is the slow dog, the last dog. Eta tells Zo he wants to take Joe for himself. The man kicks Joe with his shining boots, smacks him with his belt.

We pile into the car, topple on top of each other, pushing our sacks underneath, snarling and snapping, drooling for the smell of each other, the smell of the blood, and then Eta goes for Joe.

The man watches in his rear-view mirror, his eyes flash beneath his shades. Eta has his mouth on Joe dog's throat; all of us shriek, excited, all of us want this big dog's heart. "Heart, heart, heart!" we shriek, and Rab is going wild, but Zo grabs Eta by the hair, throws him into the bulletproof glass on the window. The man swerves, watching. He is watching and watching, hoping and watching, but Zo has become angry now, and Eta is scared.

At the man's place, we fight each other to devour the

meat he throws in our kennel. It is not much meat, less than usual.

Joe pushes forward and forward, rips a piece out of Rab's back. Eta's teeth glisten like wet stone, he and Ot go after Joe. They could kill him if Zo said, but the man is watching, the man is smiling and standing behind the mirror watching, and Zo will not even let them take Joe's eyes.

"I have plans for my little friend," Zo says. We wonder what Zo will do. Joe drags a piece of meat to the corner, hides it away, swallows it whole.

"Important plans," Zo says. He is mysterious, his mind always scheming. When the man turns off the lights, Zo's eyes still shine. All night long, we tired dogs sleep, but Zo never does.

In the morning, Eta is missing. We call and shout for Eta, sniff and scratch for him, cry for him, but he does not answer, he does not return.

Then we are back in the man's car and Eta is gone. We tumble and tangle, nip and growl, as the man rips through the city, down black side streets and jagged alleys, out to the places the rich people live.

We are fast today, even Joe dog is fast, we tear through the houses like flames, smashing safes, collecting gold, money, jewels, dragging sacks over fences, through hedgerows, to the man, the waiting man, whose teeth are like full moons. He kicks us only a little today, feeds us a little more. Joe dog does not grovel, he does not wait. He lunges for the food, the first dog, and Zo will not let us have him, he will not let us take him. We all wonder what Zo is up to, what he will do, but he does not take Joe for himself either, he does not take Joe at all.

In darkness, he nudges other dogs away, makes a sleeping place for Joe beside him.

"Lick my feet," he whispers to Joe dog. "Treat me like a man." The sloppy sound of Joe's wet gratitude bounces from the walls, and we all wonder what Joe will do for Zo.

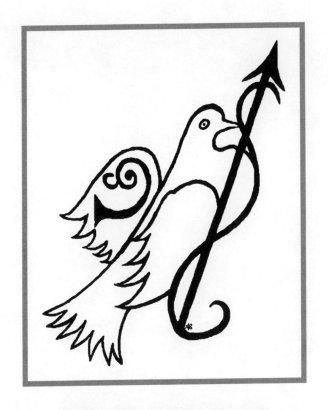

# ENCHANTMENT

**S**he remains in the shack in the forest, because he put her there, because she is afraid to leave, because he might return, and she does not want to stop hoping. She remains in the shack, watching the forest dance outside the bleak green walls, watching through an open knothole, a perfect circle.

There are young conical pines with furrowed bark, with reaching needles; the entire forest vibrates, nothing is still, and she waits, watching from her knothole, because she expects to see him, she hopes to see him fighting his way towards her.

Will he be carrying her arms when he comes? Will he have aged? It could have been a decade since last she saw him. Will she recognize him? Will he care for her? These are her thoughts that twist and twine like plants and multiply like fungus.

Her armless stumps drip blood when she is sad. "He won't come," she tells herself. "I will never see him again." Tears slide into pallid cheeks. She tries to recall the last time she saw him, running from the forest, heading away from her. She reviews the scene again, sears it in. It burns when she breathes, when she thinks, "He was angry, he swore," but then she remembers he said he would bring her arms.

Her face revives. "He will come back."

Sun rains into the musty shack. She settles in the centre of her dwelling.

"How long does it take to retrieve a pair of arms?" It feels as if she has waited forever, although she cannot be sure. In the forest, time does not exist. Days roll nights to morning.

When she stands she is clumsy. She thinks of her wounded body, feels the pit of her stomach. Slowly, she moves against the walls and with her lips takes in sawflies and tip moths, the swollen ends of inch-long termites that burrow deep canals in wood. Her tongue absorbs them and when raindrops strike the shack, she pushes her tongue through the perfect knothole and collects them.

Sometimes she sees animals in trees: racoons and rabbits, bears and deer. Sometimes they walk right up to her shack, so close she could almost touch them with her tongue, almost taste them, but they do not remain close for long. Their noses twitch and shift, she wonders what they smell, how they vanish into green.

One day, there is thunder splitting through the trees. Fallen needles jump. There is a crack, old trees snapping, the rush of panic preceding a stampede. Animals tear

through the rugged pass, deer leap wildly through the
pines.

Outside something like a man moves. She tilts her head,
presses her eye close to her knothole, considers the figure,
looks for her arms. It is not him; it is another man she sees, a
man whose hair is yellow fire.

He limps when he walks, yet his feet move as lightly as
soft fern. He bends, surveys the markings on the ground,
examines the trees. Over one shoulder, he carries a quiver of
arrows, over the other, a gun, and she wonders if she should
call to him, let him know she watches, or if she should still
her breath, quiet her hope, let him vanish.

He sits on a rock, so close to the shack she can smell his
breath. Her face warms as light spills from his open shirt,
from his mouth, pooling at his feet, touching hollows of
moss.

This man is not a man, he hides his wings. He stands,
stretching his arms, opening his hands, and her voice leaps
away from her into the tops of the conifers. He is the one who
will find her, the one who will keep her from being alone.

He is surprised. He wonders if some animal is trapped in
this crumbling edifice. He lifts broken planks, snaps thin,
rusting nails.

*Enchantment*

Her eyes lose their centres. She fights to see. His eyes fasten around her. He has never seen such a sight before, never come across such an animal. Filthy, covered in cobwebs, yet beautiful; moss grows like jade between her toes.

He orders her to stand still, not to fear him. He examines her closely. Touches the thick mat of hair on her head, looks at her shoulders. "Arms," he says. "Did you ever have any?"

Her shoulders weep.

Already he has torn his shirt to bandages. He moves deliberately over tree stumps, slippery rocks. He lifts her with his own arms, carries her over fallen debris, rotting boards. She barely notices his limp, barely notices his feet touching the ground. The bright world spins. What was it she waited for?

Beside his arrows, his gun, she hangs from his shoulder like a pelt.

Her bandages contract, the heat of him warms her. He carries her from the forest. Everything burning in his light, the shack melting out of sight.

She has no arms. She cannot wave goodbye or lift her head from his hot back to watch the forest disappear.

"We're going the wrong way," she tells him, but her

words slide to the ground. He hears nothing but the sound
of his own heartbeat, his own footsteps, as he carries them
both towards town.

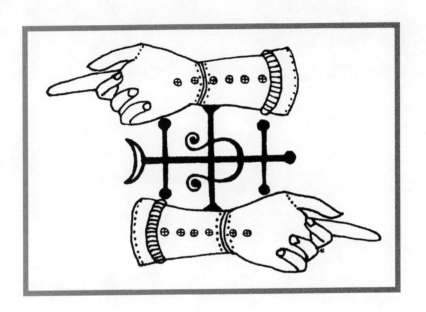

# ARMOURY

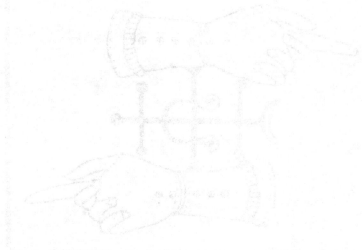

ARMOURY

It looms like a rearing monster of mirrors. Her chair rolls down its ramp. It eats the groan of metal, the sweat of fear. His flawless hands push her past the seamless walls. She cannot cry over her missing arms. She is wheeled to the chamber, the lair of this beast. Shelves pulse with treasure. A stranger approaches masked in white.

The man is jovial. "It's who you know that counts." His wink is like a wrinkle in the sun.

The stranger in a paper mask stoops to touch her wounds as if they were the only ones on Earth, as if she were the only woman. He prods her leaking bandages. "Clean cut," he declares.

She is unbound, her blood mopped clean. The stranger sutures, ignoring the blossoms of blood that collect on his fingers, the sting he inflicts.

"Another moment," he tells her, "a few more stitches." She grows excited anticipating.

The limping man touches her forehead. "Marry me?" he asks.

With arms, she will caress his shoulders, hold his hands, stroke his hair. With arms, she will embrace his brightness.

The delicate silver needle works over her wounds. Each

*Armoury*

prick is a torture, each stitch an execution, but she is anaesthetized with hope.

Ivory hands finish the sewing; they wash themselves clean of blood, they reach towards the shining shelves, retrieving arms, pairs and pairs of arms, white and black arms, plastic arms, arms of wood, chrome and silver. None she recognizes, none her own.

"My arms?" she asks. "Do you have my arms?"

"Which pair do you want?" the surgeon answers with a question. He places his collection on a table before her. He turns some to display their shapely contours, their attractive curves.

The man with the limp points to the most glistening pair. They are awkward, clunky, too heavy to manoeuvre. The surgeon eases them onto her shoulders like masks. "It'll take time," he says. "Rome wasn't built in a day." And she thinks of Pompeii, of exploding Roman candles, of heavy Roman columns crumbling to the ground.

The arms collapse at the elbow, twist like puppet legs. A burst of blood escapes at the shoulder, rolls down the polished silver expanse, drips off a silver finger.

"You'll get the hang of them," the surgeon assures. "Before long, no one will know you weren't born with them."

The silver arms groan and creak as they rise, like twin jets, convolvuli climbing complex trellises of air. She watches their heaving movement, their ungraceful pause as they reach their zenith, then clatter to her chest.

"I don't want them," she whispers.

"You're bound to feel that way at first," he says.

If she had her own arms she would leave, turn the door handle of this terrible room, escape. But the surgeon hasn't restored her and her blood runs into the silver palms of these hands. Her shoulders are packed with bright white towels, the silver needle has set back to sewing.

"You must try," the surgeon begs.

"Don't be a fool," the man with a limp echoes.

How can she accept these arms? They are not hers. Their presence only reminds her of what has been lost.

Her dripping blood is sponged away, leaving the arms bright as if polished. The needle dips and pulls, tying off eruptions, erasing the loud red. The room buzzes with the silence of silence. Her mind grows white and calm as cinder. She is led through bleached doorways and corridors, through white, blinding rooms of blood. She is taken away from what she remembers, out and away from this room. The man with a limp places a golden ring on her silver finger. "Call me

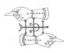

husband," he says. His hot lips seal her mouth closed and in this silence nothing bleeds.

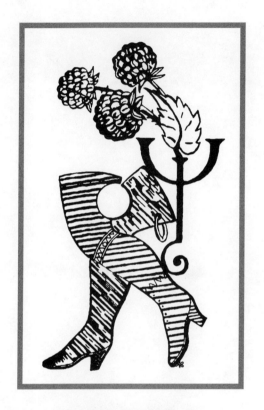

# IMPOSTOR

**H**er home is a box. Square windows on every side, soft flat grass both front and back, hedges, spiked wood gates. She teeters on her balcony, drags carpets, beats slumbering quilts. This spidering subdivision extends farther than her vision, farther than the rooftops, a chain of fallen dominoes towards the sun.

She cleans and bakes, sews clothes and curls her hair. All day long, she is busy making use of these heavy silver arms, hung like pipes from her shoulders. Now, her silver fingers slide deftly into place, move with practiced elegance over dishes, floors and toilets. They apply makeup, rub lotions into flesh, darn stockings, work out stains. Their fists punch bread dough into balls, then come away clean as fruits from their peelings. She marvels at their loneness, their ability to stay removed but ever-bright, she marvels at her own ability to use them. She wishes her husband were home to see the silver hands submerge in scalding water where they scrub the collars of his shirts. She'd like to show everything she's learned, but contents herself with making these arms so much a part of herself that in time even she will forget they are not.

When these arms have finished cleaning and cooking, scrubbing and baking, preparing for this evening's dinner party (which all day has felt impossibly imminent), she goes to her bedroom, removes her pinafore, changes. Black fabric stretches like glistening snakeskin over her naked body and the silver hands paint her face, then roll her hair high in a perfect cloud. Long white gloves unfurl beyond the edges of her dresser mirror, the silver hands put the gloves on like salve, up and over shimmering joints.

Her husband returns and is barely changed before guests arrive. She shows them into her home, pours wine, talks about the newest books, the latest movies. Her shadow evaporates like perfume, vanishes from the immaculate wall; the guests are muted by her magic, traces of her sweet scent. Her man joins her in the centre. "You're magnificent, darling," his words tangle in her hair.

"Wonderful party, superb food, delightful wine."

"Terrible headache," a woman says, cups her hands to her face, excusing herself as her eye rolls beneath a dinner platter.

In her absence, there are whispers, sly smiles, chuckles. "It popped right out of her head . . . rolled past my fruit salad like a grape! To think she could keep a thing like that to herself!"

Their giggles rise as offerings to the host and hostess.

"Unfortunate woman," he says, shaking his head.

A bearded man limps to the bathroom laughing, his leg tips like a felled tree, crashes clean from his trousers sending him into an elegant aspidistra.

"Who put that thing in there?"

There are bursts of sound. The man leans against the wall for balance, shields his empty pant leg behind a chair, and then it is as if both he and the object of his shame vanish, for the guests do not see him retreat or reappear. A woman with bright red lips and horsey teeth loses her head in the roaring jollity; it bounces, then rolls beneath the table like a bowl, her arms search to find it, to reunite it.

Mischievous feet kick the head, it rolls towards the south end of the room. The table rumbles with diaphonic abandon while the woman's inconsolable body collapses in a heap of mauve.

It is the hostess who finally retrieves the dented head, places it gently in the woman's hands.

"You'll hear more of this," the woman informs her when she has made her adjustments. She is neither grateful nor amused; she storms away from the dwindling party.

Wine flows. More hysterical tears are shed. The host and hostess hold everything like sweets behind curled tongues.

Later, it is the casualties they discuss and the ones who

dropped their guard. They laugh at the pretension, are indignant at the dishonesty, insulted by the denials.

"Anyone could tell  . . ." they repeat over and over again, absorbing the fading light from the window, gathering the sheens of warmth from the room.

Shadows, like delicate monsters, creep beyond their dimming threshold. The host and hostess retire quickly to bed. She drops her dress, pulls down her hair, rolls off her gloves, changes. He unwraps himself from his perfectly pressed ensemble, exposes his mahogany chest, his rigid armour, his golden leg. Together they shiver like lonely leaves, their brightness failing to contain the final sparks of day. They whisper into darkness, their uniqueness, their pre-eminence. "I'm sure they couldn't see your arms."

"You didn't limp."

"You held the glasses steady."

"No one could tell."

In through the window night swims like a dark shark, gobbles what little remains of their bright disguise. He closes off his mind, stops thinking. She wonders if she really is as good as she might be. That night they both dream of houses exploding, of roof shingles ripping through air like knife blades, of arms and legs, heads and torsos, shattering into oblivion. In the morning a shameful puddle of blood in their bed is avoided. He spends a long time in the shower. She finds it difficult to lift a frying pan, to crack an egg. They say nothing to each other at breakfast; he does not say goodbye when he leaves.

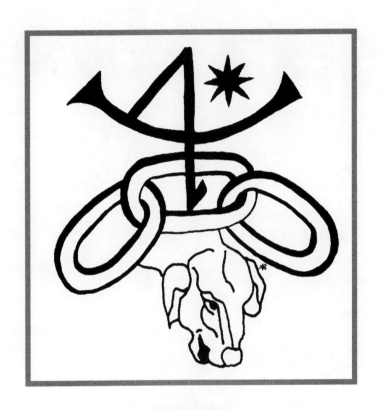

**TAKEN**

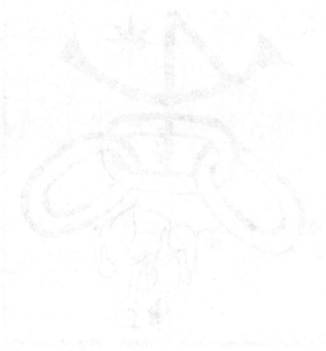

**H**orace McCutcheon is in jail. His dwelling is now free. It was something about income tax, parking violations, speeding tickets . . . something about red tape, about forgetting a zero, forgetting a date, ignoring a summons.

He didn't rob the houses after all. He didn't beat old women unconscious, maim their children, poison their talking birds. He never actually murdered anyone himself, never actually took any money with his own hands.

For all intents and purposes, by all standards of the community, he was an upright citizen, a business man who believed in the philosophy of reciprocity, the philosophy of washing, of scrubbing backs, of philanthropy: "You do for me, I'll do for you" was his motto, his trademark, his prayer.

He took in homeless boys, picked them up off the street and gave them a place to sleep, a purpose in life. It was his mission to train them, to make them productive, to give them a chance. They came to him like dancing rats, just as if he were the Pied Piper. He offered them food.

At times they lived in an underground chamber hewn from stone. As a child he had always loved caves, imagined himself a caveman, hoped these boys would also find wonder in the dank crevices of his childhood love.

It is immaterial to mention the chains, the collar braces, the piles of excavated bones and excrement. All merely props. And upstairs, what has been referred to as the kennel room – in actuality, the Ken Nel room – was named for an illustrious ancestor, Colonel Kenneth de Nel, whose father originally fled to this country from France, a persecuted Huguenot.

This man now in prison, it must be understood, came from an irreproachable ancestry. His forefathers created this country and his foremothers breast-fed it. Yet he, Horace McCutcheon, the product of a staunchly supportive parentage, somehow knew an orphan's misery, loneliness and despair. He knew an orphan's needs, and took in homeless boys, knowing their anguish, knowing their desire for discipline, for simplicity, for food.

"There are only two paths you can go," he would tell them, "the path of good and the path of evil, the right path and the wrong path, the path to your future or the path to hell." Unfortunately, the boys seemed consistently to choose the latter, in spite of his best efforts. In spite of the food.

The boys became rebellious, quarrelsome, violent. They became abusive, disgusting, hateful. Still, he didn't like to give up on them. He didn't like to turn them away. He transformed the Ken Nel room into a quiet place without noise and windows, without furniture and distraction, a lullaby room, a nursery, where the boys could think things through, find a new perspective, reflect.

The man now in jail, did not rob the houses, he did not scrawl four-letter words across the walls with blood and shit, he did not deface the family photographs, he did not rape the old men, brand their virgin daughters with fire, eat their hearts. He took the boys on outings, fit them in his car like one happy family, all in the back seat together. And when they arrived at their destination, he let them free just as if they were at a summer cottage, and they ran. They ran high into the rich suburban neighbourhoods and Horace waited patiently in his car. Some evenings it was so beautiful there beneath a purple sky it felt to him as if he had always straddled two worlds, two futures. He smoked a calming cigarette, cleaned his immaculate nails with a toothpick, hummed a little song and thought happy thoughts. Sometimes he would wait until the stars appeared; he would try to identify the constellations, envision the bull and the bears. He would think about early man, Neanderthal, and imagined what he must have thought, seeing the bright sparks of heaven appear in the sky all at one time.

The boys burned trails up the hills, they tore houses from

their foundations, juiced them of blood, made the world shake. Nothing but degrees of silence echoed from these wounds, nothing but impermeable night. They gathered money, jewellery, portable TVs; they strapped them to their backs, hoisted them over their shoulders, carried them downhill.

He put out his cigarette, blinked his eyes. The boys forced their way into his car, they crashed and bullied, pushed and smacked.

"Two worlds," he thought, and then he thought about magic, about the power of naming, the power of being in control. He thought of the magic of saying a thing is a thing, of making others believe you. He looked at the constellations and sighed.

The boys settled down on the way home. Only a couple injured. Teeth marks in bloody flesh. They always sorted things out themselves.

He fed them as always, and as always they were aggressive and rude. It is not important where the meat came from. It is not important the size of the portion, the quality, the cut, the way it was cooked or not cooked, the way it was served. What is important is that he fed these children, these outcasts, these orphaned untouchables. He gave them shelter, he gave them advice, and he gave them food.

They fought like barbarians over the meat. At times they behaved scarcely human and it sickened him to watch. It sickened him to stand behind his double-sided mirror and witness them destroy each other. He lamented their behaviour, blamed himself. Some nights, alone in bed, he wept. Some mornings when he unlocked the Ken Nel room, whole boys were missing. He didn't like to cause a scene, create animosity, accuse anyone. Negative attention produces negative results. Better to let it go, drop a veil, pretend he didn't notice, start things fresh.

How could he report the missing boys? None of them had proper names. None of them remembered their families. Sometimes it made him feel as if he'd imagined all of them, as if he'd dreamed them up himself. At times, he considered, it was like the kind of happy dream that suddenly turns bad.

"Two worlds," he mumbled. The boys grew more hateful. They obeyed him less. Their faces grew wilder, they growled and snapped at him, and he began to wonder what exactly he had done.

He wanted to let them go, wash his hands of them, make a clean start. But where does one go to abandon the

*Taken*

abandoned? And then he would feel such a sudden wave of indescribable emotion welling from his belly, climbing through his spine: guilt or panic, greed or sorrow. He didn't know. He couldn't say. He only knew that he must continue to shelter the boys. He must continue to feed them.

The Ken Nel room became for the boys a world in which only the laws of nature prevailed. There was no civility, no serviettes. They drooled and scuffled, fought and ripped each other apart.

He watched from his double-sided mirror, feeling goosebumps rise on his flesh. He was horrified, appalled. He couldn't turn away. The one who was most vicious, the one who came to rule, watched the man watching. It appeared the one who came to rule could see through walls. He could put his voice into other people's minds, read their thoughts, control them. He got the other boys to follow, got them to do everything he said. This is why the man was eager to be rid of him.

Of course, Horace McCutcheon went through a litany of pros and cons, he spent hours soul-searching, days indecisively deliberating. Could this boy be saved? In some ways, he might even be useful. However, in the best interests of the others, for their safety and well-being, he concluded the one who came to rule must go.

He had no intention of murdering him, no intention of harming him in any way. In fact, when he saw the others tearing off his face, breaking his limbs from his body, when he saw the others devouring his torso, he did not feel relieved. Only splinters of bone remained of the one who came to rule, yet the man could not feel happy. He sobbed until he collapsed, slept a fitful, painful sleep, dreamed momentarily of a lost, inaccessible world. He moped through the following day, fed the boys without pleasure, took them for their run.

Even the purple sky did nothing to cheer him, for he realized that soon another boy would come to rule, and then another, and another, and that each would grow increasingly more controlling and nothing he could say or do would ever change or override this.

The boys shoved and elbowed their way into the car. They kicked each others' groins, smashed each others' faces. They stacked their booty to the ceiling. The man could take no pleasure. Dry blood crusted their lips, sat on the tips of their fingers, stained their clothing.

Perhaps it was the howls they made, the way they fought,

*Taken*

the smells of blood and drool or just the disquieting revelations of the future he contemplated. The man drove too fast. He exceeded the limit. A bright flash of light captured this transgression.

He did not pay the speeding ticket. He did not obey the summons to appear in court. The world in which he found himself living had somehow come unmoored from the present.

Stars glittered like winking eyes in the purple sky. He imagined letters forming words and words forming phrases. "It is what you believe. . ." the heavens told him. "Rough, rough, rough. . ." he read. Slowly, he spun himself like an ebbing top, under the brilliantly sequinned sky, then carefully lay himself down on the earth: "Pay up, you bastard . . ." he read. "Give in . . ." His eyes closed, then opened again. "Fuck off . . ." the heavens finally told him.

He grew more depressed, more careless. In parking lots, he could no longer differentiate between spaces for the able-bodied and those for the disabled. Tickets piled up on his dressing table. Fines and court summons went unacknowledged. He began to slink when he walked, hide in strange places. Finally, the government began to investigate, his business was audited.

He spent hours in front of the television, his head propped in his hands. He began to neglect the Ken Nel room, began to forget to bring food. His car remained in its garage and magnificent purple evenings went unattended. Houses up high in the hills remained intact. People began, reluctantly, feeling safe.

The boys howled like hollow wind-struck caves. They roared like restless chasms. The man did not watch them fight. He did not watch them devour. He turned the volume up on his TV, flicked channels, watched talk shows and soaps.

When the police kicked his door in, he sat still on the couch as one shocked, paralyzed. Black test patterns reflecting from his eyes, his pupils rolling like tiny silver ball bearings.

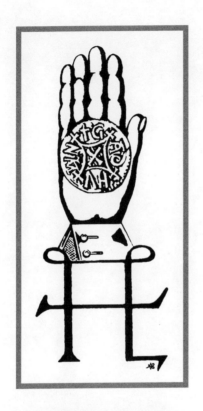

**A MAN I AM**

Joe lopes along the sizzling city streets, hightails it past courthouses, bolts and scampers through alleyways. Trucks and people appear the same to him: wild aimless arrows shooting forward into his line of vision, into his path, and so he avoids them, turns from them, rushes away like a skidding top.

Buildings stud the landscape like dangerous spikes. Joe catches himself on corners, gets sucked into the glistening, whirling doors of glass, tumbles out again upon the cold flat surfaces of stone.

Women walk quickly past him. They hold their purses tightly to their chests and canter by. Men glare at him before they cross the road.

He weaves and wobbles, tips and topples, but no one helps him to his feet, no one will approach him, for he may be violent or diseased, crazy or drunk. He may be dangerous, and people do not take risks.

Cars and buses race past, the air grows thick as oil. Joe chokes, then sputters, sprawls into the street where he would gladly remain if it weren't for the honking, the murderous raging, the oblate, ugly mouths that hiss and spit. He crawls onto the curb, rolls over the pavement. Sticky black gum,

*A Man I Am*

dirt, gravel, stick to his shirt. He rises on trembling legs, feels pain in his festering thigh, recalls where he's been, remembers his hunger.

The man who gave meat sits in his mind, Zo twists in his belly. He wants to forget both. Drool overflows his mouth, drops to the earth. He gnaws on fire hydrants, parking meters, tires. He eats a Styrofoam cup. A man's broad face expands like sponge above him. A man's pointed foot swings at him. Joe is quick, it does not graze him. He leaps away into the alley, not knowing if he should follow this man or not.

Joe feels the nerves in his aching thigh burn as he watches the man vanish into a building, and then decides to follow. The building is cold, smooth; Joe brushes against it, searching for the scent of food. He pushes his nose against its window and finally edges his body through its door.

Vests and suit jackets, trousers and ties, hang like ornaments from golden rods while all along the walls, crisp white shirts observe their splendour.

Joe sniffs the soundless air, he follows the man to distant counters, he tastes the merchandise, finds it bitter.

"Gettoutahere!" a voice explodes. Joe jumps, scampers, hides behind a golden rack.

Thick strong hands collect him, toss him in the street. "No dogs allowed!" The heavy door whispers shut. Joe stands on the balls of his feet, he stands on his toes. He peeks into the store window, watches the man he had followed sporting a new suit, the man with the frightening voice, smiling.

"I can be a man," Joe says. He brushes the splinters of broken glass, of dirt, of gravel from his skinny legs. He slides his thin trembling hand over his scalp, then licks his palms to wipe the whirls of filth away that stain his face. Two men are talking in the store. Soon the man in the new suit leaves. He enters the crowded street. Joe has no compulsion to follow. "I can be a man," Joe says.

When the other man, the man with the frightening voice, retreats, Joe seizes the moment. He goes inside. There is nothing to taking a suit, nothing to dropping the tatters of cloth that hang from his body like cobweb, nothing to finding his way inside of the suit or becoming a man. He analyzes his image, brushes his hair again with damp hands. Now he will be a man, he tells himself, and no longer be hungry.

Outside the pavement buckles with men. There are many, many men, Joe observes, and he does his best to

*A Man I Am*

emulate them: their walks, their casual greetings, their aloof disregard. He stands on the balls of his naked feet, cranes his neck from the new suit's collar, holds his shoulders high as flagpoles.

There is a gentle twinge in his thigh, a hollow rumble in his stomach. "A man," he tells himself, "a man, I am." He struts, he strides, he gazes ahead of himself, beyond himself, he fills his chest, his stomach with smoky air. The drool that threatens to collect on his lips he shoots like a bullet onto the road. He will not allow himself to feel hunger, not allow himself to be a dog.

He twists his head as he walks past windows, mimics interest, feigns disdain. Then suddenly his heart gallops, beads of perspiration slide from his brow; in a glistening store window there are boots. Tall leather cowboy boots with steel at the tips of their pointed toes. Saliva fills his cheeks, old hunger bites his belly, he spits into the street, glides into the boot store, lifts the boots with a skilful reach. On his feet they are just like velvet slippers, but they are black and tall and smell of dead flesh. He marvels at their ability to hold him closer to the sky, their power to please him. He kicks a building with a pointed toe, watches small squares of brick crumble like dust.

"I could kick this building down," he thinks and feels his body growing larger.

On the street corner in a small café, people congregate for coffee and doughnuts, sandwiches and soft drinks. Some wait outside on plastic chairs in the haze of foggy sun, squinting and fidgeting. Others collect food, carrying it back to large buildings. As they scurry past, as they beat the pavement with their flying feet, Joe notices coins that now and again drop from their pockets and roll in an arc like silver wheels. These people are not aware of their losses. Their heads do not move from their rigid gaze. Joe slides his hand next to the earth like a magnet. He draws silver to his palm.

"A man needs spending money," a voice says.

Joe thinks he will run, tear through an alley, flee from the street.

"Don't be scared," a smiling man tells him. His voice is smooth, kind. "Finders keepers," he says.

The man lingers, though Joe does not encourage him with talk; he follows Joe down the street, taking pleasure in his deft routine.

Joe continues to gather, he continues to bend and stoop and draw the shining circles to his grasp.

*A Man I Am*

"I'll buy you dinner," the smiling man offers. "Meat and potatoes, roast beef if you want."

Joe's mouth twitches. Saliva grows heavier than glue on his tongue.

"A nice rare slice of beef," the man continues, "just what a man like you needs. Let me buy it."

Joe empties his mouth of its secretions, feels his stomach painfully contract. "Why?" Joe asks.

The man extends his broad palm, he wants to shake hands. "I could use someone like you."

"I'm not a dog," Joe growls.

The man steps backwards, withdraws. "Of course you're not." Joe combs his ruffled hair, straightens his lapels, wipes again the places on his face where dirt shadows his masculine expression. The man relaxes, smiles his friendly smile, leads Joe from the sidewalk to a restaurant.

The meat the man orders is red and juicy. Joe eats all there is then licks his plate clean.

"I have a job for you, if you'd like one," the man says.

Joe feels a twinge in his thigh, a quick contraction in his craving body. Joe gnaws on his plate, nibbles his juice-stained serviette.

"A man needs work to eat," his host says.

"A man, I am," Joe answers.

The host chuckles, lights a cigarette, turns in his chair. Crevices like rock flaws mar his marbled face. He picks up the bill, counts his money, stuffs what he owes under a glass.

Outside the restaurant the pavements relinquish their heat. Joe and his host make their way down glowing streets past retreating people who move together in formation like birds flying home.

Numbers hang like ornaments from large desolate buildings. One of these buildings belongs to the man, and he takes Joe inside to show him its workings. Rows of men and women in crisp white shirts stoop over their desks scratching figures with sharp grey pencils, buzzing like insects on their adding machines.

The man is explaining something to Joe, about this business, about the job he has in mind, but Joe's thigh spasms, his stomach gurgles and demands to be filled. He can only think of the meat he has just consumed, of the spit collecting in his throat, of his desire to end his hunger, and so he says yes to the man. He tells the man he will take the job.

The man is pleased. He shakes Joe's hand. "Glad to have

you on board," he says. "I know a man like you will do us credit."

Joe swallows his saliva, wipes his lips with his sleeve. "A man needs work to eat," Joe says.

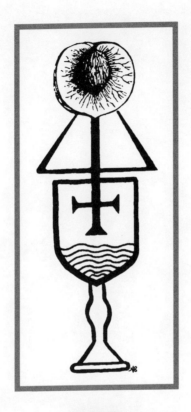

**RED**

They have stopped talking now. Run bone-dry. Words like water, which politely dripped from their lips, have finally ceased. They avoid each others' faces.

He is late coming home. She forgets to cook dinner. The parties they planned are indefinitely postponed. Bright feasts and sparkling evenings give way to gossip. Suppositions fly like random birds. She does not clean house, bake bread, mend stockings. Colourful pallets of makeup collide in a jumble of unwashed shirts. Her bed is unmade, her clothes infested with moths, and the arms that hang from her shoulders no longer glisten.

It was the blood, he said, that drove him away. Smudges of her blood, like stencilled roses, on walls, and chairs – everywhere, in fact, that she touched. In the end he could not move through the house without becoming stained by her blood, nor could he stop her bleeding.

She tried to hide it, tried to clean it up, but even neighbours strolling past could see the stains, the bright roseate markings, the flags of her shame.

Alone, she would consider her life: her exploding childhood and the house that shattered, severing the arms she imagined still swaying somewhere lightly in the trees. And in the moment she became determined to retrieve them, blood would ooze, smack the floor like sap, glaze the furniture.

Using false names she went to the best clinics, but their pills and plasters, syrups and sutures, could not heal her. "My husband," she sobbed to the doctors. "My arms!" Blood puddled in the palms of her silver hands like liquid poppies. "Neurotic symptoms," the doctors concluded, sending her home with small paper prescriptions, psychiatric referrals, assessment appointments, all marred with the hectic disgrace of her blood.

No one could help her. No one could save her. It was in her mind, this obsessive yearning. She exhausted the world with her failure.

"Why don't you help yourself, just a little?" her husband demanded. Blood rose to her shoulders like milk to swollen breasts, shot from the sleeves of her shirt, gushed in a steady fountain about her.

"You sicken me!" he muttered.

She didn't know, at first, where he went when he left, if he was going for an hour or forever; and the heart in her chest convulsed, the floor grew red. And then she discovered the photographs, stacks and stacks of photographs, hidden at the back of his closet, concealed behind his spare iron leg.

She needed a dishtowel to remove them without leaving her mark. Sordid Polaroids, all the same woman, poses of long, naked arms.

"I've tried," he finally told her, but her shoulders had already begun dripping. His face contorted as he turned away.

There was a scent to his leaving, a trace of something incendiary and a reek of decay that brought curious neighbours milling and gawking, each glance forcing a slow rising tide of red past the window ledges, each comment coating a corner, laughter lashing an entire wall.

Blood filled the house, past skirting boards and curtain hems. It swelled, leaving pink markings on ceilings, signifying the highest crests of the waves. She divested herself of tarnished, heavy arms and the neighbours watched the blood rise beyond her throat and nose, hoping it would drown her as she bobbed, a prisoner, until the large plate glass window shattered under pressure, propelling her on a slick red swell to the street.

"You think she'd have the decency to keep something like that to herself!" muttered neighbours, satisfied and disgusted. "She never was one of us," others agreed. "No arms!" shouted others. And those who once attended her parties and had basked in her perfect silver light formed a circle around her and watched her squirm, blood-soaked and armless, attempting to rise.

Without arms, she was off balance. Without arms, she could not push herself from the earth. She wriggled like a red worm, finally found her feet and fled. Children chased her, pelted her with pebbles, and the echo of curses resounded in her head. She had no idea what she was doing. No idea where she might go for help. No idea if help was what she wanted, but her feet and legs propelled her, they carried her unsteady body away, they took her to the heart of the city, and then suddenly stopped.

Between two towering buildings, beside a sanitation bin, she found herself standing in a pool of her own blood. Insatiable starlings swooped the skies above her, dipped to tarmac roads, ripped up pieces of furry animal flesh, then perched on awnings and windowsills, intrepid with their bounty. She felt a pain in her chest, a sudden, forceful constriction, and worried about herself, blood swelling from her shoulders, pumping to gutters, running through streets. People walking past slipped and skidded, recovered themselves, moved forward. A man, then a woman, then a young girl, sailed past, the soles of their shoes stained, footprints leading away from her, crazy paisley designs extending out in all directions.

She stood in the centre she had created: a rusty statue, a spike, an armless, grieving exile, thinking someone surely would help her; but after several hours she began to walk.

The streets were thick with cars that bellowed and honked and screeched, tore around crumbling corners, slowed at stop signals and exhaled balloons of grey smoke. Thinking of her husband, the pictures, the stain, she choked a little as she passed them and wondered if it was too late to go home. Could she ever make it clean? She thought of her real arms, her flesh arms, swaying, open-palmed in the trees, and then the silver ones she had abandoned.

She came to a small square park, littered with plastic cups, paper wrappers and unseemly grey bags that tumbled across patchy yellow grass, stuck to hedges and fencing, tore loose and scattered across pavements and streets. Stone garbage containers, dilapidated benches, patches of concrete scabs spotted the park, and a few meagre trees swayed, overshadowed by apartment buildings and banks.

She found a place to sit, a bench beneath a jutting iron pole, ravaged by graffiti but unsoiled by food or excrement, and noticed that the spill from her shoulders was lessening, that her depleted body was in need of sleep. City sounds, shrieks, explosions collected in the park, and she dreamed of a man who consumed the flesh of boys. All her dreams were nightmares, yet her sleep was restful. She had hoped not to rouse, hoped her sleep was eternal, but when the moon rose and the day's warmth vanished, she shivered awake. Sluggish shadows tumbled from buildings, crawled to the park, rolled out from the hedges towards her tired, trembling feet.

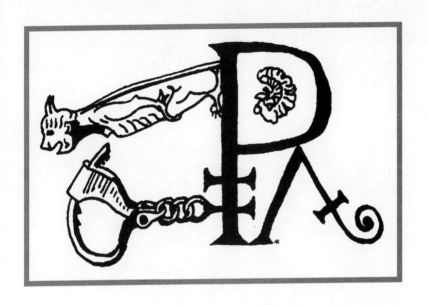

# NIGHT CRAWLERS

**W**hen night comes, we leave the building, jump down zigzagging fire escapes, push out doors. All day our mouths are busy talking. What we're going to do, the bullshit they throw at us. Markey practices golf swings in corridors, smashes windows with those bright yellow balls. He collected them all on hunting expeditions, every one he turned up a nugget of gold. He could have sold them back to the country club, could have got a dollar each, but he found an old putter in the alley, picked up a nine iron in the junkyard. Now the whole building's a golf course.

He slams those little balls through holes in the walls, bounces them off fractured ceilings. Plaster dust sprinkles our heads like powdery snow and he shouts, "All right! Did you see that?" And we nod and go back to our talking.

Water still runs in the bathroom urinals, Val rinses her hands, takes a piss. We bitch about collectivity, about people who think like cows, about ass-kissers, brown-nosers, sell-outs. If it weren't for them we'd have it made, but we stop talking at night when we hit the street, we stop talking and scatter.

Val is paler by moonlight, her skin is luminous, it glows; she has not eaten for a long time and tonight she's searching, her bulging eyes probing, her moist lips assembling.

We smashed the mirrors in the building, smashed the tinted glass. None of us could stand not seeing what we looked like, and so we always ask each other, always say.

I tell Val she's pretty, and in a waifish kind of way she is. Her long bony fingers rake her hair, and when we pass a restaurant she has the confidence to do what she has to do and grabs a total stranger's hand.

The two of them walk into an alley. I drop behind. Once, some bastard pinned her to bricks, beat her so badly she couldn't run; now I hang back, think about tomorrow, try to ignore the snuffling and grunting, try not to see what's going on.

When she comes back she seems brighter. "That wasn't too bad," she says. "I'm okay." And we stroll down the avenue, past the restaurant, past a hotel. Fog rolls from clouds, there's a patch of cobblestone, a church. "We should be wearing capes and riding horses," she says. "Everything's suddenly old."

And it's true, it seems as if the world has grown two hundred years younger, as if we are walking some foggy, ancient street, as if we have somehow stepped through time, wound up in a patch of past, a place we don't belong.

"Jack the Ripper, Mr. Hyde," she whispers, "don't be surprised if they're my next picks."

She laughs at herself, at her lightness, at the fact she has survived every murdering night. Sometimes, I know, she wishes she hadn't, and I want to tell her she's not alone. But we never talk about our options, never talk about death. It's a kind of superstition, a fear. If we start talking about it we won't ever be able to stop. Every breath will ingest it, every thought summon it, every moment contain it.

Val skips away from me, suddenly playful, swings around a dim, ornate lamppost like Gene Kelly, lands smoothly on her knees. "Closing time at the bars," she announces, "and now for my second performance . . ." A man stumbles out of the fog, weaves a crooked path towards us.

"Sir?" She stops him, grasps his jacket with her wasted hand and takes him into the heaviest mist.

I shut my eyes, try not to think or listen. The noises of her breathing, the grunting and gurgling. I cover my ears, walk away.

Sometimes I would like to keep walking. Walking and walking. I would like to walk to another place, start fresh, forget Val and Markey, the building we live in, its broken, boarded windows. Go someplace different, someplace warm, and I wonder if I continue walking if Val would find me right away or if she and Markey would have to search for me. I wonder what I'd tell them when I was found, if they'd trust me, if our lives could continue as if nothing had happened.

Val emerges from the thickening fog, eyes like glistening marbles. Her mouth is wet. Damp wisps of thin hair curl around her face. "I did him," she tells me. "He's done." There's a kind of excited hiccup in her voice, a crazy joy. Her wide empty eyes dig into the next man. She carries him off to a parking lot, finishes him in less than a minute. On her way back, she picks up another. Each time she takes one she grows stronger. Her eyes lose their innocence, her face swells pink. Soon she's snatching men, dragging them into open alcoves. Any person passing might see, might call the police.

"Enough," I tell her. "You've done enough!" She resists when I hold her, struggles to break free.

"It's hell to start, but when you're really doing it, it's like you can't do anything else. Like your car's stuck in drive, you've got no brakes." This is how she described it once. Now she can't talk about it, can't think about her greed, and I take the handcuffs Markey gave me from my pocket and fasten them on her wrists.

She cries, howls, spits in my face. "How could you . . . you bastard . . . you cow!"

She hadn't expected the handcuffs. I hadn't expected to use them.

"Talk to Markey. This was his idea." My words vanish in her tirade. She hates me, she'll never forgive me, even later when she's thinking straight. I want to run. Leave her on that foggy street corner chained to herself, swearing and raging. Instead I put my hand on her shoulder, try gently to lead her away.

Her feet scuffle on the pavement; she kicks at me and I dodge.

"Markey has the key," I yell. "If you want to get loose, find him!"

She swings at my head with her handcuffed wrists, paints the night with hate. "You fucked-up asshole jerk." She thrashes and kicks, turns my flesh violet.

"Calm down, Val," I say, though I know it's me who needs to stay calm. I jump away stinging, heart pounding, stomach twisting. She's out of her mind, way beyond reason. "We'll find Markey." My voice is deliberate, cool. If I left her now, if I ran, I wonder what my chances would be. Could I explain it to Markey if he found me? "She was crazy. She took off. I tried to catch her but she slipped away, I fell on my ass . . . see the bruises? Markey, Jesus, why did I have to use the handcuffs?" And if I got away, if he didn't find me, where could I go, how could I get there? One day he might just show up. One day he might just arrive. Wherever I went, wherever I got to, I'd always be thinking of Markey and Val.

Somehow, I manage to get behind her, loop my right hand through her bony arms.

"We're going to Markey," I tell her. "He'll set you free." And she cries like a dying gazelle because of the handcuffs, because of what she remembers, because she hates Markey and she can't kill me. I yank her along the cobblestones, make her walk to the other side of the street. The fog lifts and we're someplace else. The buildings are harder, sooty. Bars and restaurants are stained and stinking. Puddles of puke and piss collect in rockeries, window boxes, potholes. "Keep moving, Val. Pick up your feet!" She makes her body go limp, refuses to help me. The occasional smoky car passes, a limousine, an empty beer can tumbles from a windowsill, rolls past our feet.

"*Nice lady!*" a man shouts from the darkness. "How much you want?"

Val twists her head towards me, lunges for my throat.

"You can have her," I want to shout. "Take her right now!" And I wonder if I sold her, turned her over to this talking ether for money, if we'd be any happier. But then I think of Markey, feel his impatience. He's waiting in the park, tuning into our minds, searching our thoughts. I think of shocking pink lightning, a field of snow, a sunrise I once saw when I was small. "We're coming, Markey," I say in my mind, and drag Val down another city block.

At the intersection we can see the park. It glows like a spaceship with its saucer lamps. A rusting iron fence surrounds it, unkempt shrubs shrink into its shadows. Markey paces at the gates, trails back and forth.

"About time," he shouts as I approach. Val's heels dig into tarmac, her body resists.

"Why did you make me use handcuffs?" I ask him.

"Fuck off," he answers, reaching for Val.

Markey is stronger than I am. He lifts Val with one hand, holds her in the air for a long time, just as if she were weightless. She squirms like a hooked fish, tries to hit and kick, gobs at Markey's head. He blows it back in her face. When she gets tired, her body goes slack. He drops her on the pavement, takes the key from his pocket, offers to unlock the cuffs. His mind is on other things, something he's spotted, so he will not prolong Val's torment; he will not force her to endure any more of her deadly memories, the handcuffs, the craziness. He will take them off, elicit her help, and although she hates him she'll do what he asks.

The scent of blood surrounds a woman huddled on a park bench. Markey is quick to determine her usefulness and Val is dispatched to see. Bright, friendly, unnaturally warm, Val listens to the creature's story, nods, touches her with quivering hands. Markey and I eavesdrop, wait.

Markey slicks his fine hair with spit, I tell him he's handsome. I adjust my clothing, tuck in my shirt, hide the gouge in my jacket Val put there. She's telling a story, telling the woman how we came to live where we live. "We were blown apart, knocked out, now we don't fit in. We're not like people. It's bad luck, really. We've suffered for it." The woman sighs, faint vermilion circles appear at her shoulders. Markey's excited, we emerge from the darkness, stand in a circle of light.

Val is good at pretending, good at concealing our plans. "A happy coincidence," she reports to the armless woman. "Now you can meet them, now you can stay with us."

The woman does not resist, although there was no talk of this. "You must come and stay with us. Say that you will,"

Val is insistent, her eyes like knife points. "We can be like sisters, like very best friends."

Markey is charming. I smile at the woman. Her face is as empty as a starless sky. We lead her through maniacal streets, take her to our collapsing building. "Casa Condemned," Markey quips. A brimming red overflow rises and subsides at her rim, she scales the sloping stairs, brushes concave pathways with her light, frightened feet.

Val shows her to the bathroom, the urinal. She takes her to the corners of our rooms. "You can pick the place you like best," Val offers, "make it your own." But the armless woman, already asleep, her body a question mark, curls where she falls and Markey applauds.

"Can we make her love me?" he taunts Val. "Beginnings are such beautiful things. Do you remember ours?"

Val's hands make symbols of infinity. "There's nothing to remember."

"Women are fickle," Markey smiles, collecting his putter from dead electrical cables. "But who can live without them?"

Val turns from Markey. I see her hesitate, then retreat. I follow her without speaking down fire stairs, under sagging beams and broken rusty canopies. Her stride is adamant, this time she'll get away. Her hands slap the heavy door. She hasn't thought things through, hasn't considered the consequences of the hour. Dawn pours acid into the building. A streak of yellow singes her face.

"Condemned!" she shrieks, the hopeless painted message falls to her feet as she slams the door shut. Her flesh burns, she laughs at this sign, this assertion that tells her what she already knows.

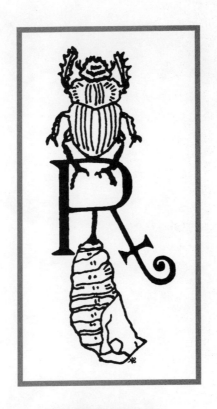

**OPENED**

All young phantoms arise this way. The blemished walls throb with them, the crooked floor where you know they'll bury you oscillates. Nothing you can do will stop them. Sun or moon or lamplight filters through. "Arms," says the vapour.

You remember stumbling through streets, slipping up asymmetrical stairs. A woman you recall, a Val or Valium, leading you along and the men, two men, one like a shadow, appearing after she spoke, absorbing your reason.

The ledge of darkness, the lonely place they left you, where your eyes became narcotic, where ancient insects scuttled from the crevice with flat oval bodies, wings they never used, rakish antennae.

You followed them, their manoeuvres. They trusted you, it seemed, deposited their eggs, let their soft white nymphs harden brown on your body. And the vapour spoke and said, "You're special," and you began to think perhaps this was your love story.

"I think I love you," the vapour whispered and you began to hope the vapour loved you. And if you could have spoken you would have told it, "I love you," because now you were sure this was your love story, because you were sure it could only love you more.

In your mind you begin to talk to it. "An explosion," you say, and wait to feel its interest billow, wait to hook the spark and fuse of its spinning love.

"An uprising?" it asks and turns your eyes to the trees that appear just ten feet from the house of your childhood. "An insurrection?"

"A vivisection," you whimper. "Two tiles off the roof of our house stole my arms, that and my parents' tar-black annihilation."

"Go on," the vapour tells you and you imagine that you hear your voice telling him about the trenches and foxholes all around the house of your childhood, that you tell him about the glittering diamonds of splintered windows, sandy roof shingles scattered like cards. You hear your parents continue arguing, smell the smouldering disdain, and your brother – you see your brother running like an injured beast away into the world. Did they know you escaped? Did they try to find you?

"Arms?" the vapour says and your vision dulls.

"In the trees," you mutter, "my arms are waiting." And the vapour whispers it would have liked for you to embrace it. It would have liked for you to be whole. It could have blown up buildings for you, dedicated itself in your service.

"I love you," you say weakly, wondering if words have emerged from your lips, if the vapour has heard you. Then you listen, hoping for clues. There are murmurs and cracklings, buzzing and gulping. You work to open your numbed eyes, work to discover your love story, but before you are able, the vapour speaks. "I never loved you," it says. "I never loved you, but I wanted to keep you."

And you think to yourself, because you no longer have the strength to imagine yourself speaking, "If you wanted to keep me, you must have loved me in some way."

The vapour is restless. "I never loved you. You were nothing to me." These words float to your ears like small dead fish and wash away.

"If I had truly been nothing, you wouldn't have to say it."

You sense the wall alive with life, with tiny bodies scattering away from light, pushing deeply into crevices, existing only on dust.

"Nothing," the vapour pulses. But you know it is the vapour's reassurance, you know it is the fulcrum of his power, you know that vapour also has no arms, and so your lips keep silent.

"Can she hear?" You know it thinks you're hollow, it thinks your mind has been sucked dry, yet it whispers anyway, it whispers and buzzes like insects whenever it passes, whenever its face turns towards you, whenever it speaks of what it is that must be done.

You are silent when the vapour travels your edges, silent when it speaks.

"Arms," it says. You dread this proximity to death, but delight in discerning this knowledge. You cling with your weary mind to your riddle.

Your lover materializes, draws you to where you find your arms happily hanging from his hands. "Take them, quickly," he tells you, but they vanish as you move. The riddle opens before you.

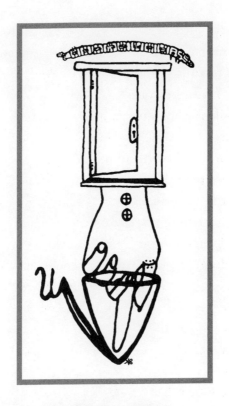

**ARM KEY**

**H**e called her Scarlet. His small joke. Not knowing her name he laughed, not knowing, but saying such things: "She's perfectly 'armless." Then, again he would say, "She completely disarms me." He spoke in soft tones to her, held her in sleep. "What do you call the coat she once wore, the coat she lost?"

We looked at each other, looked at the cockroach marching in the spiral of her ear.

"It must be her coat-of-arms," he snickered, pleased with himself, slapping his midriff, licking moist lips.

And when we complained, when we knew it was dangerous, when she had become a pillar of cloud by day, of fire by night, we begged him to bury her, begged him to put her out.

"Armageddon," he bawled. "Get it? Arm a gettin'?" He curled double with hysterics, laughed till his eyes filled with pus. "Afraid of everything," he accused us, "afraid of *this?*" Her body was stiffening in the corner, whiter than plank. Her shoulders secreted black blood at the stumps, thickening to resin. "Completely 'armless," he told us, "trust me."

We met in the bathroom. He tended her bleeding. We silently ranted about necessity. "Holes in the flooring!" We knew how to make them, how to dig with our hands in the cellar's clay.

"Distractions!"

"Errands!"

"A timely explosion!" We nodded our heads, stuck our fingers in the urinal till they crinkled, showed him our hands when we returned.

"Just a bit of cleaning," we said. He didn't make us take it further. He was busy fanning her. Busy keeping his revolution alive.

We whispered in darkness, buzzed like electric bees, crept down to the cellar, planted his explosives in the yielding clay.

We knew he was saving himself, knew that he had planned on destroying the world. "No one will take anything from me again," he had once said, and we laughed as we buried his dynamite.

"Her favourite novel?" he quipped. But we didn't understand him, didn't know what he wanted us to say. Our dirty fingers crawled behind our backs. His twisted mouth turned ugly.

"Think!" he commanded, so we bowed our heads.

The floor was rife with centipedes and spiders, fat inky-blue beetles.

"*Farewell to Arms!*" he shouted, his black wet tongue spilling over his sparkling white spears. Our feet scuffled, we wondered if we should run. He threw his head back, thundered his senseless howl. By morning, he was feeding again.

We signalled each other and crept away. The cellar was shallow. We crawled on our bellies. Crawled with our mouths full of slimy clay. We didn't expect he'd miss us, didn't expect he'd give us a second thought. We dug until our hands were drier than birch, dug until our nails shattered, our knees damaged and chunked with clay.

The smell of it became our essence. We bathed in the urinal, washed out our hair.

"He'll know what we've been doing." I didn't need to say it. "I guess we should prepare to die."

We pasted angel smiles all over our faces, tucked wounded hands into our sleeves. We tried not to limp as we followed her blood to the corner, tried not to appear petrified.

He was writing his name on the wall with her blood. "Mar-key," "Ar-key," "Arm-key."

"I never loved you," he whispered.

And we saw that her body had become a black stone, her leathery face deific.

"I never loved you," he repeated, "but I have needed you." And black blood mingled with tears and dripped like oil from his chin. "No one will take anything from me," he sobbed. "No one will take anything again."

We considered Markey wailing, knew he would never be free and couldn't help but feel sorry for him.

While we yanked up the floorboards, prepared the hole for the passing, he rambled and ranted about his armies and armchairs, swearing it all had been inevitable.

"I never loved her," he wept desperately. His eyes were hollow. He couldn't see us. And when we approached her, her chest expanded minutely with her breathing, her body emanated heat.

He cried out often in frustration from beneath the floorboards because he could not see us and we would not understand. "I am the Arm Key!" he insisted, "but I never loved her," and at nightfall, after the explosion, we left the building to find ourselves another home.

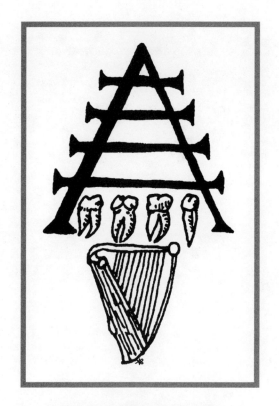

**NUMERATOR**

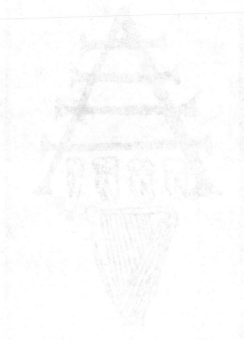

It is a dark room at the end of the hall in a building that
ticks. Numbers flash on walls, bright, neon green digits
blink on screens, flicker on calculators and adding machines.
The room hums like a chorus of drums, people scratch pulses
with pencils.

Joe is a raw recruit here, "the new man," they call him.
He's given a place at the front, a pencil of his own. The
machine on his desk spits numbers.

His pencil is newly sharpened, it carries the scent of
something forgotten. It slides over paper like grey lightning
forming perfectly oval *0*s, crisp *2*s, delicate *5*s. Joe is
mesmerized by his pencil, entranced with his ability to
command it. He examines his level *1*s, his onerous *8*s.
He turns his page upside down to determine the variation of
curves in his *6*s and *9*s. Every number announces him.
Every count asserts his pride. "I am a man," he thinks, his
shoulders rise, his backbone straightens. Printed numbers
erupt from his machine.

Scarcely in this hub of industry does his stomach's
gnawing compulsion distract him, nor does his stinging thigh
absorb his concern. His hands and eyes fill with numbers, his
mind quickens to its chores. This merging and separating,

this coagulating and reducing, this forming and transforming bewitch him. Five- and ten-digit numbers combine, and then he subtracts a two. His hand trembles. His prolific number machine heaves millions and he stabs his ledger with something new.

It is painless, this dividing, this subtracting, for nothing ever really gets amputated – nothing real ever gets taken away and nothing demands additional space – the numbers do not force him to forget or remember, and so he relaxes into his operations.

The boss paces close to Joe's desk, his face extends. Joe's heart gallops, his breath accelerates. "Good man," his employer offers and Joe must stop himself from panting and drooling, from wagging his ass, from being a fool.

He pulls himself higher in his chair, clears his throat, furrows his brow. "I am a man," he asserts to himself, "a working man." He collects ribbons of numbers accumulating on the floor, smooths them before him, summons his calm.

All day, all afternoon, Joe adds and subtracts, adds and subtracts. Crystals of graphite smudge his fingers, his face. He refuses breaks, refuses lunch. The barrenness of his belly falls numb. At the end of the day a whistle blows. Other workers flee but Joe remains; numbers and numbness hold him. His mind continues counting even after his body's collapse.

For days he works this way, waking and sleeping, increasing and reducing numbers, bound to this room of his manhood, this job.

His employer observes him, endorses this binding, but thinks that in some ways it could be improved.

"You're an excellent worker," he says, "managerial material. But a man needs a home to go to, a shower, a wife. He needs to wash his face."

Joe's tired eyes curl, his sour suit rumples, his wagging ass drops. He sets his pencil down and raises the palms of his hands to his tongue, wipes graphite from his cheeks.

"When did you last eat?" the boss asks. Joe consults his deadened stomach. Images of meat flood his thinking. "A long time ago," he says, not wanting to recall.

The boss smirks, nudges Joe's shoulder with a loose, friendly hand. "You're no good to us dead," he chuckles.

That night he takes Joe home and introduces his wife and daughter. They show Joe the powder room, give him a fresh bar of soap, a clean towel. They set an extra dinner plate, prepare the guest room, welcome him into their fold. Joe does not slaver over the dinner meat, he is careful to appear cool. The daughter beams at him. The wife passes green beans and mashed potatoes.

"Help yourself, Joe," she sings. Her voice is high and empty, charming and merry.

"Just one of the many joys of married life," the boss announces, grinding a sinewy piece of beef between his molars, grinding it to pulp.

Joe is afraid to eat, afraid to activate his slumbering hunger. "What if?" he wonders, imagining the most humiliating scenes. He notices the daughter appraising him, her corn-silk hair, her milk-white teeth. Light glints off her glasses. Drool accumulates at the back of his throat and he tries to think of numbers, of 6s and 9s, of straight level *ones*, of anything that calms him.

The daughter unfurls his serviette, pours him water, adjusts his plate. She smells of honeysuckle. Her face is always in his line of vision, always in his gaze. He's afraid she will spot his weakness, see his hunger. When he takes the meat into his mouth he's afraid he will lose control.

The daughter is solicitous, she says she knows what it's like to be new, to be a stranger, to feel self-conscious, to have people look you up and down. She tells him she knows what it's like to be shy, to want to make a good impression, to

have people like you, and how upsetting it is, how
frightening it can be, to think you might do something
wrong.

Joe thinks of numbers as he chews and the daughter's
talking puts him at his ease. Even if he were to make a
blunder, get carried away, swipe meat off someone's plate,
pinch flesh from the hostess, the daughter would continue
talking.

Throughout dinner the daughter talks, she talks about
weather and music, about the school she attends. Her parents
listen to her prattle, they enjoy it, encourage it.

"Myra's going to make some lucky man a good wife," her
father says winking at Joe. Myra's pale, freckled skin turns
strawberry, she laughs like a starling. "Don't embarrass me,
Daddy," she pleads.

When the meal has ended Myra clears the table. She
brushes Joe's arm. He is relieved the meal has ended, happy
he remains undisgraced, hopeful the worst is over. The boss
offers Joe a cigar and although Joe has never smoked, he
takes it. Myra wheels a harp into the living room at her
father's request, tunes it with patience.

"You're in for a treat," Myra's father tells Joe and ignites
the cigar with a heavy gold lighter.

Clouds of pale blue smoke engulf Joe, roll over his head, make him reel. Myra's hands sweep the harp strings, her voice rises in song and for a moment Joe is caught in a memory of childhood unconnected to himself: a ragged house, something black churning on the stove, fractured furniture. He doesn't know where these thoughts come from, why they visit him at all, but in seeing them he is doubly warmed by his present harmony, his employer's paternal care, Myra's eagerness to please.

A restlessness that's long possessed him falls back on its heels. He sinks deeply into a flowered armchair, exhales putrid smoke, allows himself to be pleasured.

Myra's voice is mellifluous, her face angelic, her presence celestial, and Joe holds her in his vision.

"It's going to be a special man who wins my little girl," Joe's employer says. His voice reverberates over the music, over his daughter's fine sound, "A man with a future, a man who'll make her happy, who'll provide for her."

Joe thinks about his future, about his manhood. He wonders about this family, this comfort, this joy. For the first time in a long time there is a sharp, gouging twinge in his thigh, a pain that resonates in the pit of his stomach – familiar emptiness. He wants this music, this harp, this voice. He wants this soft armchair, this blue swirling smoke, this busy clatter in the kitchen. He wants this father, this mother, this daughter, this house and all these pleasant feelings; he wants these things for himself, he wants these things to fill him.

Myra's glasses slip, she glances at Joe as she plays, as she slides the glasses up the bridge of her nose. Her smile is friendly, her alert body emanates communion. Joe feels easy in her presence. He feels understood.

Myra's mother brings coffee, Myra completes her serenade and before Joe knows it, he and Myra are sitting alone together on a loveseat.

"I want to help people," Myra is telling him, "I want to do good. I want to work with children or sick people or people who live on the streets. I want to go somewhere I can be useful, fight malaria or leprosy. I also want to get married. I want to marry a nice man and have children, I think. Children are a big consideration. There are so many unwanted children in the world, so many starving children. Maybe adoption is the answer. But that would depend on my husband. What do you think?"

Joe nods, feeling free to decline an answer, yet easy enough to express his opinions. He has never thought of children before, of himself as a father, and now as he does the

ripping pain in his thigh returns, images of raw meat, of
erupting blood, of violent explosions. "No children," he says.

"Of course, I wouldn't really want children, I wouldn't
really want to adopt. Perhaps I'd be happy teaching children,
teaching in a school far away from the house. Well, not too
far really, not so far that if I was needed to be home I
couldn't get there quickly, but far enough that the children
wouldn't be a bother at home. I think teaching would be a
good occupation. I think teachers are useful. And when I get
married and my husband goes to work, I can go to work too.
That is, of course, if my husband and I agree on it. What do
you think? Would you want your wife to work as a teacher?"

Joe yawns, warm and peaceful. He stretches his arms, too
lazy to think. He would like to sleep, he would like to crawl
in between the soft flowery sheets that cover the guest room
bed. He would like to close his eyes, to dream, and in the
morning find himself surrounded by this warmth.

"I'm a very good cook, by the way," Myra says. "Did my
father mention that? I cook very well. Do you like to eat?
You look like the kind of man who does, not that you're fat
or anything. Gosh no, you're skinny, but I'd like my husband
to be a kind of skinny man who I could fatten up. Would you
like to be fattened up?"

In the last few minutes Joe has grown so lethargic, so totally restful, that he can no longer follow Myra's flow of words. His eyelids droop and he startles awake, time and again, each time with Myra speaking.

"Of course I wouldn't really have to fatten up my husband. I would just want for him to be healthy. You know, eating from the major food groups, getting plenty of exercise and rest. Would you like a wife to do that for you, or would you consider that nagging?"

When Joe no longer moves, when his eyes are completely closed, she nudges him awake, offers to find him a toothbrush, leads him to his room.

"My mother says bachelors neglect themselves. She says they eat poorly and don't get enough sleep. Is that true? Do you like being a bachelor?"

Joe follows Myra through the house, thinking. He has never thought about being a bachelor, never considered himself in this way.

At the threshold of the guest room, Myra leans towards him. "You can kiss me if you want," she offers. "Would you like to kiss me?"

Joe has never kissed a woman, never pushed his lips against anything but food. Myra's full mouth pleats, her lips

*Numerator*

contract. She nudges forward, quick as a hummingbird, grazes Joe's mouth with her own. There is a small electrical charge, a sudden jolt of hunger.

"A girl can't be too careful," she says. "A girl needs to set boundaries. At least that's what my mother says. My mother says that men find it hard to control themselves. She says men will always try to push a woman further. Do you think that's so?"

Joe smiles vacantly, he anticipates the softness of his bed.

"You can kiss me again sometime," Myra offers. "Maybe next time you can kiss me twice. That is, if you want to. Maybe we can go see a movie. Do you like movies? There's a good movie always playing in town. You can take me to see it if you like. I'm sure my parents will let you. You can take me tomorrow night. Will you be staying a while?"

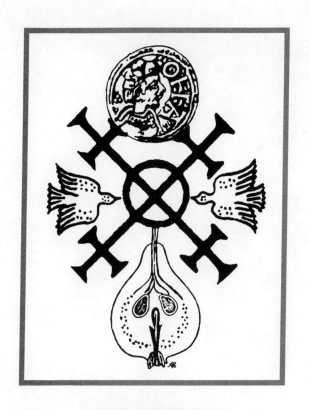

# FRACTION

In the spring Joe and Myra are married. They move to a starter home two blocks from Myra's parents, four blocks from Joe's work. Joe's boss and father-in-law co-signs their mortgage. "Joe's a good man," he tells the banker, "a good employee, a good son."

Every morning Joe walks to work; he puts in eight full hours, sometimes more. Myra packs his lunch, cuts crusts from his sandwiches, fills his thermoses with soup and coffee. Joe eats quickly, thoughtlessly, between sums. He ignores hunger, ignores food.

At the end of the day Myra waits for him. Sometimes she walks to his building, sometimes she lingers at home. She has made the home nice for him, planted daffodils in the garden, baked apple pie. She has cleaned house, organized closets, scrubbed shelves, balanced bank books, paid bills. Coupons for fabric softener, tissues, tomato sauce are neatly clipped and stacked on bleached counters. Walls have been papered and painted, floors stripped and waxed.

Joe relaxes in front of the fireplace. He drinks coffee, smokes a cigar. After Myra tidies the kitchen she joins him. She talks about her day, the high cost of groceries, the adjusting of a hem on the curtains she's made.

"It would save us money if we had a vegetable garden," she tells Joe. "Do you think that's a good idea? Of course, I'd plant everything: carrots, broccoli, cauliflower, lettuce. I could put in a couple of fruit trees too. It would be a while before we had any fruit, but fruit is so expensive at the grocery stores."

Joe yawns, listens to Myra, numbers dance fleetingly through his thoughts.

Myra pulls out the ironing board and iron, a bundle of Joe's clean white shirts. "We can talk while I iron," she tells him, methodically undertaking the task. She has sewn these new shirts for Joe, as well as a brand new suit. "My father says it's important that a man look his best . . . no creases, no wrinkles. He says you're one of the best men he knows."

Joe feels a rush of pride, a sudden peaking of ego. He likes Myra to talk this way, asks her to tell him more.

"My father says you're the best worker in the building, your productivity is second to none. He says they'll be making you a supervisor soon, and an assistant manager before long. Of course, that will mean more money for us. We'll be able to build onto the house, add a den, a sewing room, a workshop. Maybe even a built-in swimming pool, would you like that?"

Joe hasn't thought of promotions or built-in pools, he hasn't thought of additions to his house. He remains in the living room while Myra puts the iron away. She cleans the bathroom, sweeps the kitchen, vacuums under his feet. She douses the flames in the fireplace with a pitcher of water, turns down the sheets of their bed.

Joe dreams of numbers, of adding and subtracting. In the morning, after breakfast, after he has washed his face clean and put on his neatly pressed suit, he walks to work. Coils of paper twist over his wrists, wind around his feet and ankles under his desk. Machines purge themselves of numbers, hum and tick like bombs.

A grey-faced man falls forward in his chair. Two supervisors carry him from the room. His machine continues grinding and thumping, spinning out paper webs. "He was too old," someone whispers. "They should have made him leave before." They bicker and howl over his numbers, fight each other to see who'll take his place.

At night, Joe walks home in a daze, Myra sets his dinner before him. He eats without knowing, without tasting. He sits in the living room till Myra tells him it's time to sleep.

His days and nights are filled with numbers, while Myra plants gardens, builds greenhouses, constructs rockery designs.

*Fraction*

By the end of the year Joe is a supervisor, then assistant manager. He tends his own figures, monitors the progress of others, collates and compiles their tallies. Myra buys books on home maintenance, on home improvement. She orders bricks and concrete, roofing and insulation. She buys three thousand yards of electrical wire, slabs of plywood, broad wooden beams. One evening, Joe arrives home from work at midnight and discovers Myra has knocked the back walls of the house out with a sledgehammer.

She serves him a plate of simmering stew, explains she has started renovations. She works through the night with Joe waking fitfully to the sounds of squealing power saws and the smells of mutilated wood.

He dreams of a woman in black lace, wonders if it's possible to be in someone else's dreams, dozes again, thinking of numbers, willing himself to dream of work, but the dark curtains transform to veils, the room itself spins to gown.

He tries to count the spires on her coronet, the number of dark jewels on her fingers. The banging of nails, the sudden sharp grind of a sander intrudes, the woman trails into the darkness, into the walls. Myra soothes him with warm milk and Aspirin, she tucks him gently into bed. The next day on his way to work he thinks he sees the woman turning quickly down an alley.

Throughout the day he thinks about the woman, about his dream. The number machine fires paper into space, his reveries cost him productivity.

"Your mind's not on it today, my boy," his father-in-law says. "I hope that daughter of mine isn't keeping you awake at night. A man needs sleep."

Myra completes the renovations, paints and papers the new rooms, digs a swimming pool in the back. "Are you happy?" she asks him. "What one thing would make you really, really happy?"

Joe can't answer her, he hasn't thought about happiness, hasn't thought about anything that he wants or needs.

"Do you ever dream?" he asks Myra, but Myra is intent upon cleaning, cooking and canning fruit. The small cherry and plum trees she planted are bearing fruit this year. Her fingers are red with their juice. "I never dream," she giggles.

*Fraction*

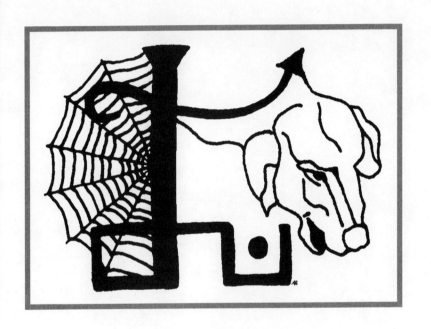

SUM

She finds you in circles of shallow sleep, touches your
wading thoughts. She is the story you learned in your
cradle, the song you were unable to sing. Her currents
overwhelm, the tiers of her hair entangle you like weed. She
is everywhere, on street corners, in hotel lobbies. You see her
in reflections when you glance away.

Your wife asks questions, wonders if there's anything she
can do. She takes your temperature, makes a broth, boils
lemons and honey in a sweating pan. She mothers you, nurses
you, swathes you in blankets. Your dark mistress stirs in your
comfort, steps from the shadows when your wife turns away.
She exposes the stinging creases of subterfuge.

The woman you've married is inhuman, your job, your
life, a fraud. It is not your thinking, but your dark mistress
shaping this doubt.

She speaks to you, beyond fiery fibres of bone, shows you
the luminous regions of your dismemberment.

Your stinging thigh combusts and hunger grows. You see
the dog you were, your eyes refuse to blink; your dark
mistress draws you deeper. There was a forest where you ran,
you ate, you slept, where you fled your first annihilation, a
house with broken walls you left behind, and your wife is

shaking you, pulling you from the dampened covers, telling you, "Count to ten."

Numbers cloud your thinking, they undress before you, tumble like acrobats over your bed. You hear your wife ask you questions, tell you things.

"It's a fever," someone says.

Your wife packs ice around your wrists, under your armpits while your father-in-law forgives you, excuses you because, he says, you've been working like a dog.

Even in trance, you resist your wife's attempts to extinguish your multiplying flames, your father-in-law's insistence that you cool. Once you would gladly have obliged them, wagged your timorous tail, thought only of the coolest numbers pouring in an avalanche of snow.

Pools of melted ice endow the air you breathe with mist, inspire your conviction, and you dive into your ancient dwelling, the place of your mistress, the home of your whole life. There was something you left in the forest, something forgotten. Your mistress lures you through the jungles of irregular pines. There was something in the trees above you, in the arrowhead ivy, in the splintering grey sheds of hobo design. But before you reach your destination, before your mistress opens the door on your future past, your wife commandeers you. She is using the garden hose she moistens the earth with. Frosty water cascades upon your chest, collects in curling rivers under your back, douses your quest, and you see her placid face, her certain cure, and you know that if it were the house, the city, the world ablaze, she would quench it.

Long after you're well, your dark mistress visits you; she joins you in your hazy morning walks and late at night when sleep eludes you she rises from your frothing sheets. You are distracted, unfocused, you do not always arrive home on time. Your boss, your father-in-law, tells you your productivity is down; he's worried, concerned about your future, and your wife asks you if there's another woman.

Your dark mistress laughs, she murmurs into her veil. That night she takes a knife and cuts your sleeping wife's hand. There is no blood, only fine electric blue wires, small fuses, silver solder. She encourages you to explore your wife's head, to remove artificial hair. You have never been this intimate, never known the plastic casing, the flesh-toned portal of your wife's workings, the embossed words that read: "Caution: never remove cover unless qualified to do so."

You confront your father-in-law, your boss, who assures you it was for your own good. He reminds you of early days, of the crumpled suit you wore, your dirty face, your sleeplessness. "Behind every great man is a great wife," he offers, and you're sure he hears your dark mistress's growl.

Streamers of numbers pump from machines, flooding the floors of your building. Your arms are heavier than iron, your mind preoccupied, your stomach sick. The numbers 2 and 4 waver before you, make faces, stick out their tongues, and your dark mistress asks you if you know where they originate, what they represent.

It is difficult to calculate, difficult to comprehend that numbers have existence beyond your sums. Your boss tells you not to worry, take an Aspirin, finish and go home, but your dark mistress leads you past ticking clocks, past disconcerted people rushing mindlessly through seasons. Numbers slide away from them, drop from coat pockets, fly from hats without them ever guessing what they lose. "The elixir," she whispers, and you know it's more valuable than gold.

On the pavement, your ragged claws are scraping, your festering thigh has made you limp. Hollowness devours its echo and into the forest, down brown needled paths, through channels of green you follow your dark mistress. She feeds you with bark and berries, comforts you with pine bow

beds and bathes you in diaphanous streams. Your memory
returns slowly; it filters through brambles and swaying trees
driving you deeper into the forest. Your twitching nose
catches a former scent, your path becomes familiar. For days
you travel, anticipating your destination, transforming your
hunger.

In the centre of a narrow clearing you find a battered
hovel that crumbles as you breathe. Ponderous moss bows its
ceiling, uprooted cedars tilt its walls. The muscles in your
throat contract, your eyes burn, boards tumble at your touch,
and the thick green world around you blackens.

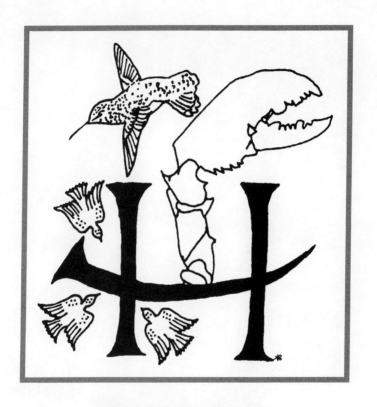

# MYRA'S ARMY

When the alarm sounds, they congregate like gregarious locusts. Some accidentally trample tomato plants, bend fruit trees, shatter greenhouse panels. Some tumble in the swimming pool and bounce like vapid toys.

They all wear pastel colours, flowered fabrics, bright pink jewellery. Their shoes are green and orange, needle-heeled, elegant designs. Overflowing to suburban roads, they throng to recognize their commander, he who assembles them, signpost stiff, clutching a megaphone.

"Daughters," he calls them. Clicking heads incline. He outlines the problem, explains the mission, slim jaws harden, he dispatches their rage.

"I'd have done anything to make him happy," she sobs, "but he left me for a shadow!" Myra is programmed for weeping, for resentment.

Her sisters buzz like angry hornets: "He shouldn't be allowed to treat her that way. Who the hell does he think he is? Someone should teach him a lesson!" Her sisters are programmed for compassion, revenge.

The commander raises his hands, silences the gathering. "Get him back," he orders.

*Myra's Army*

The daughters drone and murmur, their voices acrimoniously whirr. "Get him back, get him back." Sharp aluminum wings cut through floral coverings, engines blast, the smell of smoky fuel colludes. The daughters rise en masse and sail. Their sensitive compasses tick and twist, they flock in roving clusters, roll across the forest.

They turn the sky darker than sable, swarm into a solar eclipse. Beneath them, Joe touches wood. Filters of light scar the trees. He asks himself what mars his miracle, imagining the end of his world.

Gargantuan birds rain like angels from heaven, hit the soil about him in crumpled patterns. "Run," says his mistress, and her body breaks into tiny clouds. His feet shuffle pine needles. He's knocked to the earth. Dirt fills his mouth. He's blindfolded, trussed, dragged to the sky.

Does he remember losing consciousness, does he remember passing out? When his eyes open, Myra is beside him embroidering handkerchiefs, hooking a rug.

"You had a fall," she tells him. "The doctor says you shouldn't try to move."

His mouth is already sealed. His body inaccessible to him.

"I'll take care of you," she promises. "Everything will be fine."

His captive eyes find Myra's busy hands. Her sharp silver needles, their jagged hook-ends.

"The doctor says you might not be able to walk for some time, but daddy says as soon as you can sit, you can go back to work. That is, if you want to."

Numbers form in Joe's mind. When he can speak, he asks Myra for a calendar. He does not dream, does not think. Each day, Myra keeps track for him. "You came home three months ago, started speaking last week." She circles the days of his milestones in bright red.

He depends on her for company, depends on her for lunch and dinner. When summer comes she lifts him gently from his bed, places him in a lawn chair by the pool. Warmth penetrates his flesh. His injured back and wasted legs stir. Myra coats his body in lotion, turns him at regular intervals.

"You'll be able to sit in a wheelchair soon," Myra tells him. She rigs up weights for him, massages his legs and back each night. He counts the number of repetitions he does, the number of Myra's strokes. In less than a month he's back at work.

He doesn't remember his accident. Numbers fill the empty spaces in his history and he is grateful for his work. Myra designs a homing device for his wheelchair that transports him directly to and from her. He calculates the distance as he travels, adds the mileage every night. He counts the new additions Myra makes to the home, the number of stitches on her knitting needles, the number of plums and apples and pears on her fruit trees. He counts the days and the nights, all the efforts made for his recovery, all the transfers from wheelchair to bed. In time, he comes to count the passing years, the number of months since he stopped hoping he might walk again, the number of days he believes he might have left.

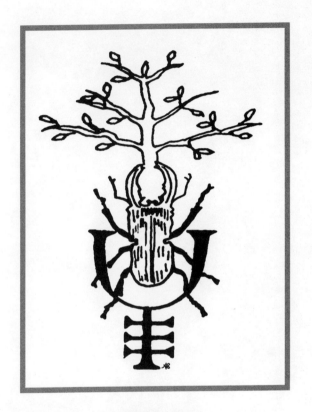

**SMOKE**

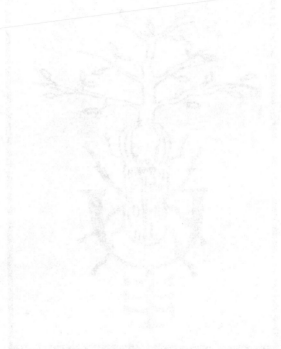

White haze crawls into her sanctum, drowns the scuttling of insects seeking shelter in her sleep. The prince has not kissed her, the curse remains. Her eyes jerk open, mysterious frames. All around is ruin. Holes as large as houses spread over the building, spewing timber and brick. She lifts her neck. Sticky black blood fixes her torso.

One detonation jarred her from death and now, feeling the warmth of the floor on her back, the slick give of melting blood, she's reckless for freedom. She wiggles loose from her adhesive bonds, pulls herself to standing. Aqua flames lick the walls, run up beams, turn orange as they touch the ceiling and her sudden breath, her sudden desperation, propels her away. She nearly floats, her naked feet grazing flaming corridors, charred stairs. Entire walls surrender in her wake and she drifts beyond her captivity, beyond her dream, out into the fierce pink rash of day.

The building is levelled, dust wells, hunks of brick, nuggets of plaster, chips of ashy timber shower the streets. Hordes gather to witness as she sails.

"She's the one," someone shouts, reaching for her blackened shoulders, her cinder hair.

"Touch my baby!" pleads a woman, revealing her baby's fractured head, the place his bones did not knit, and brains as soft and grey as down, beating beneath his bundled blanket. A man brushes his noseless, eyeless face against the blackened stains of her covering as she stoops. Legions of hands reach for the fringe of her garment, snatch up fallen crusts of her blood.

The gathering multiplies, expands. Four city blocks cannot contain it. The disfigured and feeble fall at her feet, trembling, grasping, thrusting towards her.

She manoeuvres her body through the crowd; it is uncertain, and as brittle as a shell. Hands and fingers stretch out to her and a path opens where she walks.

Trees sway and bow, undulate like dragons, lash out with sharp sickle claws. Lightning and thunder, wind and rain, force her followers' retreat, yet she advances into this chaos, into these trees that part like green jaws.

She is uncertain where to go, how to travel, but tracks and byways open to her and she finds she is lifted through this turbulent expanse. Carried back through swells and basins, past wild-leafed ferns and fanning streams. The shack that held her pierces the landscape, she recalls her longing, the despair of her shoulders. Beyond this construction lie bars of pointed ivy, bones of fallen children who lost their way. Rugged barricades of earth and mossy walls of stone yield.

She sinks in a yard, a square clay patch. The disabled house is smaller than she remembers, its fractured windows less jagged, its broken doors new and smooth. Her shoulders tingle but remain dry as she scans the roof of her former dwelling, scans the overhanging trees, searching for the objects of her quest.

Birds call, jump from rustling leaves, swoop to skim her smoky hair. Fleshy worms swinging from pine branches arrest her. The tree is larger than she recalls, fuller, and she shimmies in between the swaying green, reaches tense-mouthed for dangling fingers, for abandoned hands that crash to earth.

"Poor arms," she cries. They fold one upon the other, and she presses close to the sticky bark, alights quickly to reclaim them. Lifeless, they lie in dusty clay, ragged, weathered, pecked by jays. She examines their stunted contours, their dwarfish curves, marvels at their fingernails, toy pearls. These are child arms, small arms, too short to reach around tree trunks, too weak to lift the lightest branch. Scarcely more than infant arms, she measures. Her pasty shoulders sting but do not bleed; it is her eyes that overflow.

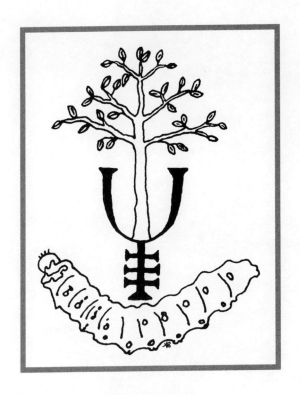

# RITUAL

My arms were the colour of cobalt, my arms were the colour of daylight. The arms of my childhood rest in this ground. I have buried them here in peace. I have sprinkled ashes over their mounds, spoken with their spirits, sang to their visions, summoned their expression. They have said: *Go write our story.*

You are two parts of one miracle. You are two parts of this ritual. I've buried my arms in these words. You the mourners. You the beholders. I have held my arms in my heart, I have held my arms in sleep. I have held my arms like my breath, in my mind and in my body. I have held my arms until death.

I hold the pen in my mouth, to put the picture in your mind.

*Tell them the arms of childhood are gone forever. Those who read these words will know, and the arms of their own childhood will be unloosened from the trees of their memory, and they will take up pens, strings and keys, while their voices spill out, and their healing will be as a fine white mist, and the creatures of the earth shall rise and cast away their wordless suffering.*

*Words are your arms,* the spirits sang.

I looked to the place of my arms and the words of this

story written. The spirits said, *And they shall hold the days of your life and the nights of your days and the years of your destiny. They shall capture all you lose.*

And the light rose beyond the sky, to the east, and the sky rose above the trees, to the south, and the rich green limbs of the trees swayed to the north and in the centre fir and hemlock extended their branches.

Emerald moss cascading through twigs, long arching boughs rounding to trunks. I saw the sorrel brilliance of the forest floor fill the centre, spores breathing from every digit of fungus and fern.

I saw the roots of each tree expand, fingers flourish through the verdant decay, through brown needles and loam, through the drying husks of pill bugs. At every direction I saw the roots extend through solid walls of clay, through pillars of pebbles, through ceilings of stone.

*These are your arms,* the spirits said. And I felt these arms open. I felt these glistening arms unfurl and I saw these words written.

*This is your ritual and these are your arms, and all those who read these words may carry from them this tuber of healing, knowing that these small, lost arms, now mourned and buried, sustain us as flesh sustains seed. We know that these arms endure, as trees endure, and grow beyond scars*. And the spirits of the arms said, *There is nothing lost*. And the spirits of the arms remade themselves in these words.

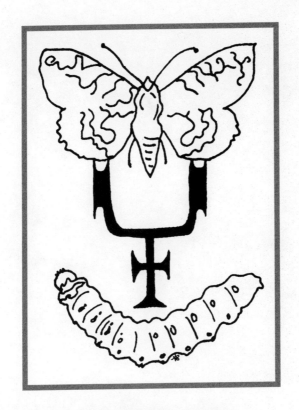

**AFTERMATH**

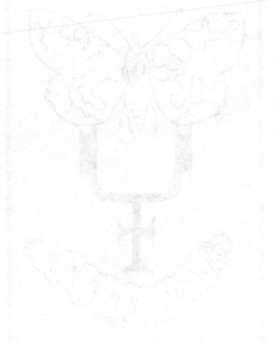

It has begun raining. Sheets of water curtain factory windows, solid streams of fluid find their way into resolute holes. Myra has dressed him securely, a rain poncho, waterproof pants. She has placed him in his wheelchair, set him on his way. He rolls along the sloping sidewalks, splashing waves into the street. His plastic goggles steam, rivulets of liquid fall from his hood. He cannot count the raindrops that land on his lap, they cluster together before they drain off, creating puddles in his plastic covering.

But this rain, this strange rain, crawling under his collar, slipping down the curve of his spine, quenches his desire to tabulate. He is aware of its feeling, its form, aware of a hunger. His chair takes him into an abandoned flooded street, jolts, skids, comes to a halt. He expects the chair to start again, but the rain prevents its moving. The rain lashes his face, drenches his skin. Long strings of drool mingle with rain and drop from his chin. Everyone has abandoned the streets, moved to higher ground. Upturned umbrellas float past, galoshes, briefcases, one straw hat and now a single white flower twirling like a miniature world. His eyes follow the flower, circle its helixes and travel its revolutions. His stomach moans, saliva overflows. He whimpers and dribbles, unable to snatch the flower from its watery dance. Alone, he is unable to lift his body from the swirling water and the higher it climbs, the more he is aware of his desperate hunger.

In this moment he is conscious of his thinking, conscious of his thoughts: he will rock back and forth, tip the chair, swim free. He will crawl away from this city, slither on his belly. He will eat berries and bark from trees, find wild honey. But before he can determine the best way to proceed, a voice breaks from above him demanding he stand. It demands he walk. Crying for Myra, hoping she will come, he yelps and whimpers, but it is his dark mistress who emerges from the deluge, his dark mistress returned.

She makes him stand on quaking legs, leaves him when he falls. He struggles to follow her and feels the wound burn in his thigh, chasing a fuse to his belly.

Through flooding streets he hobbles towards the forest, towards higher ground. "This is the place where you ran from your own self," she tells him.

He's lying on the ground again. Rain pelts his naked face, pushes his body deeply into the soil. "I am a seed," he tells himself. His body sinks deeper.

In the pliant yellow soil he uncovers caverns, tunnels, shafts, all familiar to his eyes as if sight has just ripened.

Worms, large and red, tangle in the straw-gold clay, they twist their elastic bodies into knots, feed on the minerals and elements, feed and excrete the simplicity of earth.

"Remember when this was our path?" I ask him. "Remember when we were blown away?"

He knows it is not his dark mistress. She is nowhere to be seen. She has led him to this clearing, left him, like a creature dead, under the muscle of mountain, under malignant pines; she has left him in a savage detonation of rain, with tunnels collapsing in upon themselves, with the sky blistering purple, and my voice dividing him from the trees.

He is alone in the earth, swallowed by the pain of the thorn that pierces his thigh and the hunger that consumes him and sounds that swing above him like fleshy vines and roots.

His eyes are voluminous blooms that will not close. His mind is unable to reckon. Fine white mist collects these words and delivers them down from the branches.

I am the girl from his childhood, a woman now, standing before him as he whimpers at my feet. In my eyes there is a place where he sees his own eyes, where he sees me reflected whole and recalls how he ran, how he tried to subtract me from the ledger of his life, tried to forget all we had shared and then could not recall anything.

We are both young and infinitely old, twisted in the slick moist yellow earth of our past, covered in bark splinters and needles. The barbed thorns drop from his thigh like buttons from a shirt, ringed circles in a puddle. In a puddle the broken house appears, the place that maimed. Deformed roof shingles litter the grass where we tunnelled, shattered diamonds form rainbows in the juniper shrubs where we hid. The house, once so large, is dwarfed by what it has done, made small by the show of all it held and all it failed to contain. Doors of fetid wood swing sideways from their rusting hinges. Windows sweat like eyes. We step through the vitreous shadows and the house of our childhood breathes. Crows and squirrels argue on its steps. Flax and pine weed, ash and thick sap perfume its air. We gather forks of green myrtle and fireweed, stitch them with shoots of grass. Inside cupboards and corners, footsteps, utterances, ghosts guard the thresholds we brush clean.

The inner reaches show places where we shielded ourselves, scars and stains, the acrid landmarks of our beginning. Walls have been removed, coats of plaster-dust cover floors and grey paint sheets drape furniture. There are stairways shut off by doors and sounds behind them we have never heard.

The rooms of our childhood are missing, kitchens and bathrooms take their place, the ceilings have been extended, closets made larger, shelves and cupboards modernized, renewed as if after we had gone they had decided to make room for us.

We follow the path of our past up the stairways, to the quivering doors, to the timbre of whispers, and hold our cold faces against these knots in painted wood. Our parents no longer reside here; they have left it for us, willed it to the ones they thought dead. The doors bluster free. There is no heat in these rooms but that of summer air, an expanse of light, and a fragrance of teeming life to caress us.

# Acknowledgements

*Arms* was originally written as a magical text of healing and as my black cord dissertation for 13th House Mystery School. I wish to acknowledge the two 13th House Wiccan priestesses who oversaw my magical training and initiated me into the Wiccan path: Yvonne Owens and Alison Skelton. I wish to thank Alison, also, for her countless readings of this work in order to devise relevant symbols as chapter breaks.

I am indebted to George McWhirter at the University of British Columbia, who took an interest in the original work, encouraged me to publish it and generously, patiently and kindly assisted at every stage of its revision.

Some of these chapters have appeared, in different forms, in *Descant, Event* and *Wascana Review*.